ALLERGIES AND INFECTIOUS DISEASES

LEPROSY

EPIDEMIOLOGY, TREATMENT STRATEGIES AND CURRENT CHALLENGES IN RESEARCH

ALLERGIES AND INFECTIOUS DISEASES

Additional books in this series can be found on Nova's website under the Series tab.

Additional e-books in this series can be found on Nova's website under the e-book tab.

ALLERGIES AND INFECTIOUS DISEASES

LEPROSY

EPIDEMIOLOGY, TREATMENT STRATEGIES AND CURRENT CHALLENGES IN RESEARCH

ROGER S. KOPP
EDITOR

New York

For permission to use material from this book please contact us:
Telephone 631-231-7269; Fax 631-231-8175
Web Site: http://www.novapublishers.com

Additional color graphics may be available in the e-book version of this book.

Library of Congress Cataloging-in-Publication Data

ISBN: 978-1-63321-668-6

Library of Congress Control Number: 2014946013

Published by Nova Science Publishers, Inc. † New York

Contents

Preface

This book discusses the current challenges in the research of leprosy, as well as the epidemiology and treatment strategies available.

Chapter 1 – Leprosy is a chronic granulomatous infectious disease that affects the skin and peripheral nerves; its causative agent is the obligate intracellular bacillus *Mycobacterium leprae*. The etiological diagnosis of the disease in its paucibacillary (PB) form still needs to be improved, because the bacillus is not yet cultivable. In the last years, the authors have introduced specific primers to detect the Ml *MntH* (ML2098) gene of *M. leprae* by polymerase chain reaction (PCR) and quantitative PCR (qPCR). They have been able to identify the bacillus in the oral mucosa of PB and multibacillary (MB) leprosy patients, considering that mucosa is the main route of bacillus transmission.

Regarding the clinical observation of seven MB leprosy patients who presented thromboembolic phenomena (TEP) during corticosteroid therapy, used alone or in association with thalidomide or multidrug therapy regimen for leprosy, the authors have evaluated whether single-nucleotide polymorphisms (SNPs) of the *β2-glycoprotein I (β2GPI)* gene contributed to the risk of leprosy and antiphospholipid antibody syndrome (APS) comorbidity in a case-control study. On the basis of the results, Leu247Val and Trp316Ser SNPs might represent genetic risk factors for anti-β2GPI antibody production in MB leprosy patients. Therefore, the criteria used to prescribe thalidomide and anticoagulation therapy must be improved when antiphospholipid antibodies, such as anti-β2GPI, exist in MB leprosy patients, to avoid TEP and pulmonary embolization.

Leprosy involves a spectrum of clinical manifestations—from tuberculoid to lepromatous poles—that correlate with host cell-mediated immunity against the bacillus. Besides environmental and lifestyle factors, host genetic susceptibility has been attributed to the clinical diversity of the disease. The solute carrier family 11 member *1* gene (*SLC11A1*), also known as *NRAMP1* (natural resistance-associated macrophage protein 1), has been described to control susceptibility of inbred mice to intracellular pathogens, including *Mycobacterium*, *Salmonella*, and *Leishmania* microorganisms. Susceptible mice are homozygous for a nonconservative glycine to aspartic acid substitution in the fourth transmembrane domain of *NRAMP1*. The human homologue *SLC11A1/NRAMP1* has been cloned, and several variants within the *SLC11A1/NRAMP1* gene have been described. Accordingly, the authors have evaluated nine polymorphisms [(GT)n, 274C/T, 469+14G/C, 577-18G/A, 823C/T, A318V, 1465-85G/A, D543N, and 1729+55del4] of the *NRAMP1/SLC11A1* gene in a case-control study. The polymorphisms 274C/T in exon 3 and 469+14G/C in intron 4 of the *SLC11A1/NRAMP1* gene are associated with susceptibility to leprosy. Furthermore, (GT)n polymorphisms in the promoter region of the *SLC11A1/NRAMP1* gene are associated with protection against or susceptibility to leprosy.

Recent studies on both innate and adaptive immune responses to *M. leprae* have provided hypotheses for candidate gene association studies. Because a comprehensive report of such genetic polymorphisms in a Brazilian leprosy sample is not available, the authors have investigated the association between the polymorphisms toll-like receptor *(TLR)-4 896A/G;* vitamin D receptor *(VDR) Bsm*I, *VDR Apa*I, *VDR Taq*I, tumor necrosis factor-alpha *(TNF-α)* -308G/A; interleukin *(IL) -10* -1082G/A, *IL-6* -174G/C, *and IL-1Ra* 86bp variable number tandem repeat (VNTR) genes and susceptibility/resistance to leprosy. According to the authors' results, genetic polymorphisms related to *TNF-α* -308G/A and *IL-10* -1082G/A may constitute genetic markers for susceptibility to leprosy and clinical outcomes.

Given the current challenge to eliminate leprosy, especially in remaining endemic countries, the authors hope their studies can contribute to new perspectives for the treatment and prevention of this disease.

Chapter 2 – Leprosy is a chronic infection caused by *Mycobacterium Leprae*. The spectrum of clinical manifestations depends on different *Mycobacterium Leprae*-responsive T-cell subsets. Tuberculoid leprosy is associated with type 1 T helper cells, while T helper 2 cells are primarily associated with lepromatous leprosy (LL). LL is characterized by intense polyclonal activation of B lymphocytes resulting in multibacillary and disseminated disease, as well as development of a variety of autoantibodies. The antiphospholipid syndrome (APS) is an autoimmune disease that is characterized serologically by the presence of antiphospholipid antibodies (aPL) and clinically by vascular thrombosis and/or recurrent pregnancy morbidity. The APS-associated aPL are mainly directed against β_2-glycoprotein I (β_2GPI) and prothrombin. On the other hand, aPL linked to infectious disorders are primarily directed against phospholipids and do not tend to be associated with the clinical manifestations of APS. This distinction, however, was found not to be absolute. Patients with LL present high prevalence of IgM aPL that bind β_2GPI, but they not develop thrombosis. Recent evidence suggests that APS autoantibodies to β_2GPI bind to critical epitopes in domain I, and leprosy-related aPL recognizing β_2GPI tend to be directed against domain V. The position of the epitope in the β_2GPI molecule seems to be critical for aPL pathogenicity in clinical manifestation of APS. It is accepted that aPL found in APS patients are themselves pathogenic. Patients with APS and those with LL show different *in vivo* cytokine profiles and circulating levels of tissue factor as well as differences in ongoing systemic coagulation and cellular activation. The most convincing support for the pathogenicity of aPL comes from animal models. In a murine model of thrombosis and endothelial cell activation the authors found that purified aPL reacting with β_2GPI from leprosy patients, in contrast to those from APS are not able to activate endothelium and to enhance thrombus formation *in vivo*. It could explain at least to some extent the different clinical behavior of patients with APS and leprosy-related aPL.

Chapter 3 – Leprosy is still a big social and public health problem in many countries. Brazil has been for years in the second worldwide position in incidence and prevalence, after India in this ranking. Among the nearly five thousand Brazilian counties, 252 are priorities for actions to control and prevent of this disease. The highest prevalence occurs in the north region due to intense migratory flows and poverty. In the Amazon 35% of Brazilian cases are notified, currently the state of Pará is one of the major representative of the region. Leprosy associated with pregnancy is uncommon, with few and old publications about the theme. The Lucio's phenomenon was observed as the most frequent association complication in the last trimester of pregnancy, when there is an increase in depression of cellular immunity. The aim of this study was to analyze the epidemiological situation of this association by counties and Integration Regions (IR) in Pará State, from 2007 to 2009. Epidemiological and socio-demographic data obtained from the database of the National System of Notifiable Diseases, of the Ministry of Health, Pará State Health Department and Brazilian Institute of Geography and Statistics were analyzed. An epidemiologic indicator was developed to calculate the

Detection Coefficient of the Association between Leprosy and Pregnancy (DCLP) also statistical and spatial analysis were performed through the percentile and Kernel methods in order to create the parameters of endemicity needed to evaluate the magnitude of the association and its distribution in each county of the state of Pará, taking into consideration socioeconomic characteristics. As a result it was observed that in 2007, 2008 and 2009 the DCLP was equal to 0,31 with 7 hyperendemic counties, 0,30 with 5 counties and 0,19 with 2 hyperendemic counties, respectively. Eldorado dos Carajás and Conceição do Araguaia, both in the southeast of the state had the highest coefficient of detection in the period (5,7 per 10.000 inhabitants) and a "very high" standard within the three years of study, respectively. Despite CDHGs have shown in most counties endemic pattern as "low" and decreasing year by year, in the studied period the unsatisfactory results of the analysis of social and epidemiological variables showed that the surveillance system has been ineffective in achieving the goal of the Organization World Health Organization (WHO), which is to reduce the prevalence of leprosy to less than one case per 10,000 inhabitants. The interpretation of the parameters of DCLP enabled the generation of qualiquantitative analysis, allowing to draw the socio-epidemiological panorama of the association, making the coefficient developed a new and useful analysis tool, because the informational contents produced may be used in planning processes and adoption of more efficient measures of surveillance and control of the disease, mitigating its social consequences.

Chapter 4 – Antimicrobial peptides or host defense peptides as defensins and hepcidin are fundamental components of human innate immunity. A growing body of recent evidence suggests they have a role in a broad range of diseases as cancer, allergies and infections, including leprosy.

Antimicrobial peptide inhibitors (APIs) are physical, chemical or biological agents that downregulate human antimicrobial peptide expression. In leprosy there is upregulation of both hepcidin and human beta defensin 3 which leads to opportunities for intervention.

In the case of the hepcidin-mediated iron sequestration, this can enhance opportunistic infections and a possible role in facilitating *Mycobacterium leprae* growth. Corticosteroid prednisolone suppresses human beta-defensins 2 and 3 in leprosy patients with type 1 reactions (T1R). However, costicosteroids inhibits the NF-κB pathway that causes immune suppression in the long term. These reactions are the main cause of nerve damage in leprosy.

Additionally, antimicrobial peptide elicitors (APEs) of human beta defensins could help to enhance the antimycobacterial response against *M.*

leprae. The challenge is to find specific and mild inhibitors as APIs that combat T_H1 inflammatory response without compromising the host immune system or use in combination with APEs of defensins. In this context, APIs and APEs could help in leprosy treatment with lessened induction to side effects. This could be helpful as a new and/or adjunctive therapy to find novel and specific APIs, APEs and/or anti-inflammatory agents in order to limit *M. leprae* growth and prevent nerve damage in leprosy patients.

In: Leprosy
Editor: Roger S. Kopp

ISBN: 978-1-63321-668-6

Chapter 1

Leprosy: From Clinical Diagnosis to Benchwork

M. J. F. Brochado, Ph.D.[1], N. A. de Paula, MsD[2] and A. M. Roselino, M.D., Ph.D.[3*]

[1]Post Doctorate student, School of Medicine of Ribeirao Preto, University of São Paulo, Ribeirao Preto, Sao Paulo, Brazil
[2]Biologist, Laboratory of Molecular Biology, Section of Dermatology, University Hospital of Ribeirao Preto, School of Medicine of Ribeirao Preto, University of São Paulo, Ribeirao Preto, Sao Paulo, Brazil
[3]Associate Professor, Division of Dermatology, Department of Medical Clinics, School of Medicine of Ribeirao Preto, University of São Paulo, Ribeirao Preto, Sao Paulo, Brazil

Abstract

Leprosy is a chronic granulomatous infectious disease that affects the skin and peripheral nerves; its causative agent is the obligate intracellular

---

* Address for correspondence: Ana Maria Roselino, M.D., Ph.D., Associate Professor, Coordinator of the Laboratory of Molecular Biology, Section of Dermatology, Coordinator of the Division of Dermatology, Department of Medical Clinics, School of Medicine of Ribeirao Preto, University of São Paulo, Av. Bandeirantes 3900, 14049-900 Ribeirao Preto, Sao Paulo State, Brazil. Phone/Fax: +55.16.3602.1522, E-mail: amfrosel@fmrp.usp.br.

bacillus *Mycobacterium leprae*. The etiological diagnosis of the disease in its paucibacillary (PB) form still needs to be improved, because the bacillus is not yet cultivable. In the last years, we have introduced specific primers to detect the Ml *MntH* (ML2098) gene of *M. leprae* by polymerase chain reaction (PCR) and quantitative PCR (qPCR). We have been able to identify the bacillus in the oral mucosa of PB and multibacillary (MB) leprosy patients, considering that mucosa is the main route of bacillus transmission.

Regarding the clinical observation of seven MB leprosy patients who presented thromboembolic phenomena (TEP) during corticosteroid therapy, used alone or in association with thalidomide or multidrug therapy regimen for leprosy, we have evaluated whether single-nucleotide polymorphisms (SNPs) of the *β2-glycoprotein I (β2GPI)* gene contributed to the risk of leprosy and antiphospholipid antibody syndrome (APS) comorbidity in a case-control study. On the basis of the results, Leu247Val and Trp316Ser SNPs might represent genetic risk factors for anti-β2GPI antibody production in MB leprosy patients. Therefore, the criteria used to prescribe thalidomide and anticoagulation therapy must be improved when antiphospholipid antibodies, such as anti-β2GPI, exist in MB leprosy patients, to avoid TEP and pulmonary embolization.

Leprosy involves a spectrum of clinical manifestations—from tuberculoid to lepromatous poles—that correlate with host cell-mediated immunity against the bacillus. Besides environmental and lifestyle factors, host genetic susceptibility has been attributed to the clinical diversity of the disease. The solute carrier family 11 member *1* gene (*SLC11A1*), also known as *NRAMP1* (natural resistance-associated macrophage protein 1), has been described to control susceptibility of inbred mice to intracellular pathogens, including *Mycobacterium*, *Salmonella*, and *Leishmania* microorganisms. Susceptible mice are homozygous for a nonconservative glycine to aspartic acid substitution in the fourth transmembrane domain of *NRAMP1*. The human homologue *SLC11A1/NRAMP1* has been cloned, and several variants within the *SLC11A1/NRAMP1* gene have been described. Accordingly, we have evaluated nine polymorphisms [(GT)n, 274C/T, 469+14G/C, 577-18G/A, 823C/T, A318V, 1465-85G/A, D543N, and 1729+55del4] of the *NRAMP1/SLC11A1* gene in a case-control study. The polymorphisms 274C/T in exon 3 and 469+14G/C in intron 4 of the *SLC11A1/NRAMP1* gene are associated with susceptibility to leprosy. Furthermore, (GT)n polymorphisms in the promoter region of the *SLC11A1/NRAMP1* gene are associated with protection against or susceptibility to leprosy.

Recent studies on both innate and adaptive immune responses to *M. leprae* have provided hypotheses for candidate gene association studies. Because a comprehensive report of such genetic polymorphisms in a Brazilian leprosy sample is not available, we have investigated the association between the polymorphisms toll-like receptor *(TLR)-4*

896A/G; vitamin D receptor *(VDR) Bsm*I, *VDR Apa*I, *VDR Taq*I, tumor necrosis factor-alpha *(TNF-α)* -308G/A*;* interleukin *(IL) -10* -1082G/A, *IL-6* -174G/C, *and IL-1Ra* 86bp variable number tandem repeat (VNTR) genes and susceptibility/resistance to leprosy. According to our results, genetic polymorphisms related to *TNF-α* -308G/A and *IL-10* -1082G/A may constitute genetic markers for susceptibility to leprosy and clinical outcomes.

Given the current challenge to eliminate leprosy, especially in remaining endemic countries, we hope our studies can contribute to new perspectives for the treatment and prevention of this disease.

Leprosy is a chronic granulomatous infectious disease that affects the skin and peripheral nerves; its causative agent is the obligate intracellular bacillus *Mycobacterium leprae.* While the etiological diagnosis of the multibacillary (MB) form of leprosy is easier to achieve, diagnosis in the paucibacillary (PB) form still needs to be improved, because the bacillus is not yet cultivable (see review of leprosy in Goulart, Goulart, 2008; Lastória, Abreu, 2014; Penna et al., 2013; Polycarpou et al., 2013; Rodrigues, Lockwood, 2011). In the last years, we have introduced specific pairs of primers to detect the Ml *MntH* (ML2098) (proton-dependent manganese transporter) gene of *M. leprae* in human samples by polymerase chain reaction (PCR) and quantitative PCR (qPCR) (Cruz et al., 2011; Kim et al., 2012; Morgado de Abreu et al., 2014).

PCR with Primers for *MntH* (ML2098) Gene Amplification Sensitively and Specifically Identifies *M. Leprae* in Human Samples

Detecting *M. leprae* is a difficult task: it is currently impossible to cultivate this bacillus *in vitro*, and it takes a long time to grow this microorganism in experimental animal models. The number of diagnostic methods available for the clinical confirmation of leprosy in routine laboratories is limited. Among these methods, microscopic assessment of lymph or tissue swab and histopathological analysis to search for alcohol-acid-resistant bacillus might not be specific enough. To detect alcohol-acid-resistant bacillus reliably, it is necessary to have 10^4 microorganisms per gram of tissue (Shepard, 1968), a factor that limits the diagnosis of the PB form of the disease and of recent infection by *M. leprae* mainly, because bacilli are rare or inexistent in these cases.

In the late 1990s, PCR and sequencing of the *M. leprae* bacillus genoma (Cole, 2001) enabled scientists to develop molecular detection methods to identify mycobacteria DNA.

PCR offers many resources that can overcome the deficiencies of other methods employed to diagnose bacterial infections. PCR can detect some copies of the target gene sequence, allowing identification of microorganisms that exist even in low amounts in the sample. Knowledge about the genome of the organism to be identified aids design of primers or probes, which ensures a refined and specific search and answers questions concerning the species, gender, and/or complex. Moreover, real-time PCR allows for quantification of the target in the clinical specimen, providing information about disease load and progression (Jagielski et al., 2014; Kim et al., 2012).

The PCR technique has been successfully used to detect *M. leprae*. It is a simple, rapid, and sensitive method to detect small quantities of DNA in the sample. Additionally, it is possible to conduct PCR directly on the collected material, dismissing the need for mycobacterium cultivation (Banerjee et al., 2008; Banerjee et al., 2011; Job et al., 2008; Martinez et al., 2006).

Compared with other methods, PCR is statistically more efficient to detect *M. leprae* (Shiu et al., 2000) in various quantities and in different types of samples, such as blood, biopsy, lesion swab, and lymph imprint (Aye et al., 2011; Goulart et al., 2008; Rocha et al., 2012). It is possible to obtain PCR positivity in lymph samples stored in paper filters even four years after collection (Smith et al., 2004). Moreover, PCR detection can be accomplished in the presence of very low amounts of *M. leprae* molecules (100 fg for conventional PCR and 25 fg for real-time PCR) (Martinez et al., 2006).

The PCR technique enables and facilitates bacillus detection and quantification, especially in the PB form. It furnishes valuable information about *M. leprae* infection and transmission, allows one to evaluate how effective multidrug therapy is in the case of leprosy, and reveals which mutations are associated with resistance to the treatment (Chae et al., 2002). Although many studies have used the PCR technique and a number of primers to target sequences in the bacillus *M. leprae*, no standard reaction exists for the diagnosis of this disease (Banerjee et al., 2011; Cruz et al., 2011; Goulart et al., 2008). Our research group has been using new primers to amplify specific internal sequences of the *MntH* gene of the bacillus *M. leprae* (Cruz et al., 2011). This gene codifies a protein homologous to Nramp (Mn^{++} and Cu^{++} transport transmembrane protein), expressed in many bacteria. This suggests that Nramp originated early during evolution. The *MntH* gene of *M. leprae* bears 37% identity with the human *SLC11A1/NRAMP1* gene. Hence, designing specific pairs of primers for the bacillus *M. leprae* is vital, to avoid crossing with the human *SLC11A1/NRAMP1* gene during the use of human samples (Kim et al., 2012).

A pair of primers proved to specifically identify the bacillus *M. leprae*—it amplifies the internal sequence of the *MntH* gene, to yield a 336 base pairs (bp) fragment. To test how specifically primers identify *M. leprae*, human and rat DNA samples, and DNA of different microorganisms, mainly *M. tuberculosis*, were used. Samples of patients with leprosy in the PB and MB forms were also employed to assess sensitivity. The PCR results were negative for identification of *M. leprae* in the samples (blood and tissue) of healthy individuals and patients with hepatitis C. They were also negative in the case of mouse samples and of *L. (L.) amazonensis*, *L. (V.) braziliensis*, *L. (V.) guyanensis*, *L. donovani chagasi*, *T. cruzi*, *M. tuberculosis*, MAC (*Mycobacterium avium* complex), and *Mycoplasma pneumoniae*. Using the *MntH* gene cloned in plasmid as control, only the samples from patients with leprosy showed amplification of the expected fragment, which confirmed that this pair was able to identify *M. leprae* with 100% specificity and 85% sensitivity (Figure 1).

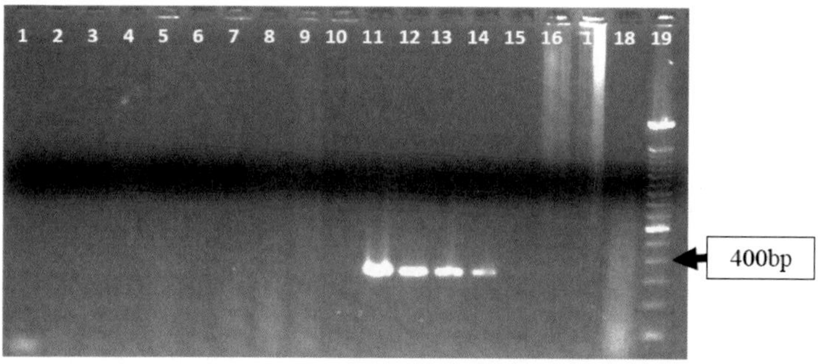

Figure 1. 1.5% agarose gel of the PCR products. 1: negative control (without DNA); 2: *L. (V.) braziliensis*; 3: *L. (L.) amazonensis*; 4: *L. (V.) guyanensis*; 5: *L. donovani chagasi*; 6: *Trypanosoma cruzi*; 7: *Mycobacterium tuberculosis* (culture); 8: mouse lung infected with *M. tuberculosis*; 9: lymph node sample fixed in formol/paraffin with PCR (+) for *M. tuberculosis*; 10: atypical mycobacterium (MAC); 11: Ml *MntH* gene 1.3 kb cloned in plasmid; 12: biopsy of mucosa from a patient with leprosy, stored in formol/paraffin; 13: biopsy of mucosa from a patient with leprosy, stored in formol/paraffin; 14: frozen biopsy of skin from a patient with leprosy; 15: imprint of biopsy in paper filter of a patient with leprosy; 17: blood sample from a patient with hepatitis C; 18: *Mycoplasma pneumoniae*; 19: molecular weight marker with 100 bp.

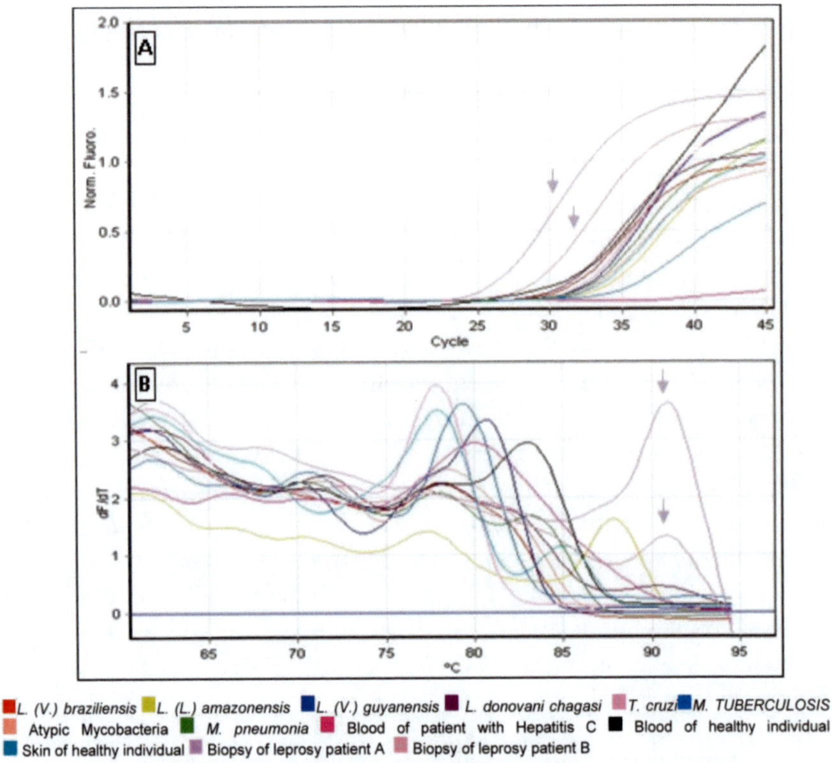

Figure 2. Specificity of the pair of primers for the Ml *MntH* gene in the various tested samples. (A) Real-time PCR amplification curve with the pair of primers for the Ml *MntH* gene; (B) Melting curve. Sample positive for *M. leprae* (purple arrow).

Conventional PCR analysis provided negative results for some samples from patients with suspected leprosy. However, real-time PCR was able to identify the DNA of the bacillus. Serial dilution of the genomic DNA of a human skin sample with positive PCR for *M. leprae* showed that real-time PCR was able to detect the bacillus DNA at a genomic DNA concentration of 150 pg/μL. Over 300 different samples from patients with leprosy (blood, frozen skin or skin in paraffin, or lymph imprint) were tested for this purpose. Depending on the sample type, results showed 22.6 and 66.7% positivity in the PB form, (Cruz et al., 2011; Morgado de Abreu et al., 2014). Together, the data showed that PCR, especially real-time PCR, was highly sensitive to detect the bacillus (Figures 2 and 3).

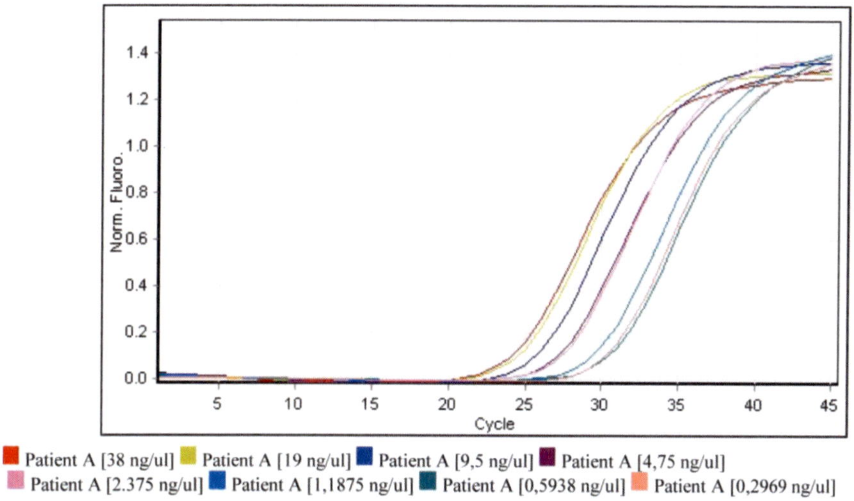

Figure 3. Sensitivity of real-time PCR with primers for the Ml *MntH* gene. Amplification curve with serial dilution of total DNA extracted from the biopsy of multibacillary patient lesion – 38 ng/μL to 0.30 ng/μL.

References

Aye KS, Matsuoka M, Kai M, Kyaw K, Win AA, Shwe MM, Thein M, Htoo MM, Htoon MT. 2011. FTA Card Utility for PCR detection of *Mycobacterium leprae. Jpn. J. Infect. Dis.* 64(3):246-8.

Banerjee S, Ray D, Bandopadhyay D, Gupta S, Gupta S, Ghosal C, Biswas N, Bhattacharya S, Dutta RN, Bhattacharya B. 2008. Development and application of new efficient multiplex polymerase chain reaction (PCR) in diagnosis of leprosy. *J. Indian Med. Assoc.* 106(7):436-40.

Banerjee S, Biswas N, Kanti Das N, Sil A, Ghosh P, Hasanoor Raja AH, Dasgupta S, Kanti Datta P, Bhattacharya B. 2011. Diagnosing leprosy: revisiting the role of the slit-skin smear with critical analysis of the applicability of polymerase chain reaction in diagnosis. *Int. J. Dermatol.* 50(12):1522-7.

Chae GT, Kim MJ, Kang TJ, Lee SB, Shin HK, Kim JP, Ko YH, Kim SH, Kim NH. 2002. DNA-PCR and RT-PCR for the 18-kDa gene of *Mycobacterium leprae* to assess the efficacy of multidrug therapy for leprosy. *J. Med. Microbiol.* 51:417–22.

Cole ST, Supply P, Honoré N. 2001. Repetitive sequences in the *M. leprae* and their impact on genome plasticy. *Lepr. Rev.* 72:449-461.

Cruz AF, Furini RB, Roselino AM. 2011. Comparison between microsatellites and Ml *MntH* gene as targets to identify *Mycobacterium leprae* by PCR in leprosy. *An. Bras. Dermatol.* 86(4):651-6.

Goulart IMB, Goulart LR. 2008. Leprosy: diagnostic and control challenges for a worldwide disease. *Arch. Dermatol. Res.* 300:269–90.

Jagielski T, van Ingen J, Rastogi N, Dziadek J, Mazur PK, Bielecki J. 2014. Current methods in the molecular typing of *Mycobacterium tuberculosis* and other mycobacteria. *Biomed. Res. Int.* 2014;2014:645802. doi: 10.1155/2014/645802. Epub 2014 Jan 5.

Job CK, Jayakumar J, Kearney M, Gillis TP. 2008. Transmission of leprosy: a study of skin and nasal secretions of household contacts of leprosy patients using PCR. *Am. J. Trop. Med. Hyg.* 78(3):518-21.

Kim OM, Paula N, Roselino AM. 2012. Cap 72 - Métodos diagnósticos em Biologia Molecular aplicada a Dermatoses Tropicais. In: Lupi O; Cunha PR, Eds. Rotinas de Diagnóstico e Tratamento da Sociedade Brasileira de Dermatologia. P. 463-71. Ed. Gen AC, ISBN 9788581140841.

Lastória JC, Abreu MA. 2014. Leprosy: review of the epidemiological, clinical, and etiopathogenic aspects - Part 1. *An. Bras. Dermatol.* 89(2):205-18.

Martinez AN, Britto CFPC, Nery JAC, Sampaio EP, Jardim MR, Sarno EN, Moraes MO. 2006. Evaluation of Real-Time and Conventional PCR Targeting Complex 85 Genes for Detection of *Mycobacterium leprae* DNA in Skin Biopsy Samples from Patients Diagnosed with Leprosy. *J. Clinical Microbiol.* 44:3154–9.

Morgado de Abreu MA, Roselino AM, Enokihara M, Nonogaki S, Prestes-Carneiro LE, Weckx LL, Alchorne MM. 2014. *Mycobacterium leprae* is identified in the oral mucosa from paucibacillary and multibacillary leprosy patients. *Clin. Microbiol. Infect.* 20(1):59-64.

Penna ML, Grossi MA, Penna GO. 2013. Country profile: leprosy in Brazil. *Lepr. Rev.* 84(4):308-15.

Polycarpou A, Walker SL, Lockwood DN. 2013. New findings in the pathogenesis of leprosy and implications for the management of leprosy. *Curr Opin Infect Dis.* 26(5):413-9.

Rocha AS, Cunha MG, Diniz LM, Salgado C, Aires MA, Nery JA, Gallo EN, Miranda A, Magnanini MM, Matsuoka M, Sarno EN, Suffys PN, de Oliveira ML. 2012. Drug and multidrug resistance among *Mycobacterium leprae* isolates from Brazilian relapsed leprosy patients. *J. Clin. Microbiol.* 50(6):1912-7.

Rodrigues LC, Lockwood DNJ. 2011. Leprosy now: epidemiology, progress, challenges, and research gaps. *Lancet Infect. Dis.* 11(6):464-70.

Shepard CC, McRae DH. 1968. A method for counting acid-fast bacteria. *Int. J. Lepr. Other Mycobact. Dis.* 36:78-82.

Shi L, Yajima M, Kawatsu K, Matsuoka M, Kashiwabara Y. 2000. Comparison of polymerase chain reaction, immunohistochemistry and conventional histopathology in the diagnosis of early leprosy in Sichuan Province of China. *Nihon hansenbyo Gakkai Zasshi* 69:147-55.

Smith LM, Burgoyne LA. 2004. Collecting, archiving and processing DNA from wild life samples using FTA data basing paper. *BMC Ecol.* April 8;4:4.

Leprosy and Thromboembolic Phenomena

The antiphospholipid antibody syndrome (APS) is characterized by the presence of antiphospholipid antibodies (aPL) in patients with thromboembolic phenomena (TEP) and gestational morbidity. Antiphospholipid antibodies consist of anticardiolipin antibodies (aCA), primarily lupus anticoagulant and anti-β-2-glycoprotein I (anti-beta2GPI) antibodies, and they react against plasma proteins bound to phospholipids or against negatively charged phospholipids (Brochado et al., 2009; Brochado et al., 2010; Pierangeli et al., 2007).

Since 2000, de Larrañaga et al. have demonstrated that anti-beta2GPI antibodies of the IgM isotype occur in leprosy patients; indeed, these authors found positivity in 29 (57%) of the 51 patients that they studied. Following this study, aCA, anti-beta2GPI, and antiprothrombin antibodies of the IgG and IgM classes were quantitated in 176 untreated leprosy patients, to show that the levels of IgM anti-beta2GPI and IgG aCA were significantly higher in the lepromatous leprosy and multibacillary (MB) patient subgroups (Arvieux et al., 2002).

Anticardiolipin antibodies (aCL) are the primordial aPL described in syphilis, and many other viral, bacterial, and parasitic infections have been shown to induce aPL. Whilst aCL frequently occur in viral infections, particularly in HIV (49.75%), HBV (24%), and HCV (20%), it is very rarely associated with anti-beta2GPI and is not correlated with risk of thrombosis or hematological manifestations of the APS (Sène et al., 2008).

Antiphospholipid antibodies, such as aCL and anti-beta2GPI, are present in MB leprosy patients; however, MB patients do not usually present with APS. According to the literature, aCL often occurs in leprosy (42.7%), where it is frequently associated with the presence of anti-beta2GPI (44.8%), but not with thrombotic events (Sène et al., 2008). In contrast to APS, increased levels of aCL and anti-β2GPI antibodies occur in leprosy patients, being IgM the predominant isotype. The frequency of aCL and anti-β2GPI antibodies is significantly higher in leprosy patients as compared with healthy individuals (15.8% vs. 3.1%). The lepromatous form predominates among aCL positive leprosy patients (Ribeiro et al., 2011).

Although authors have not identified TEP in leprosy patients, while aPL occurs mainly in the MB form of leprosy, in 1960 Rogers JH described a leprosy patient with coronary thrombosis, cerebral vascular accident, and pulmonary embolism. Since then, some case reports have dealt with this subject. Sharma et al. (2004) were the first to describe the association of deep vein thrombosis with thalidomide prescription in a leprosy patient (Akerkar et al., 2005; Bakos et al., 1996; Hebe et al., 2013; Sharma et al., 2004; Vetrichevvel et al., 2008; Yamaguchi et al., 2012). Thalidomide has been associated with venous thrombosis mainly in the treatment of multiple myeloma (Cesarman-Maus et al., 2012).

Our casuistic comprised the clinical observation of seven leprosy patients who presented TEP during corticosteroid therapy, used alone or in association with thalidomide or multidrug therapy regimen for leprosy. Therefore, we evaluated whether single-nucleotide polymorphisms (SNPs) of the *β2-glycoprotein I (Beta2GPI)* gene contributed to the risk of leprosy and APS comorbidity in a case-control study (Brochado et al., 2009; Brochado et al., 2010).

Complete DNA sequence analysis of the *Beta2GPI* gene has identified about 150 SNPs including four in the coding region: Ser88Asn, Leu247Val, Cys306Gly, and Trp316Ser (Chen et al., 2006). The mutation Leu247Val in domain V of the *Beta2GP1* gene exposes hidden epitopes with consequent development of anti-beta2GP1 antibodies (Atsumi et al., 1999).

In our case-control study, we identified SNPs Ser88Asn, Leu247Val, Cys306Gly, and Trp316Ser in 113 Brazilian leprosy patients. Additionally, we quantified anti-beta2GPI antibodies and plasma concentrations of beta2GPI. Ser88Asn, Cys306Gly, and Trp316Ser SNPs did not constitute risk factors for APS in leprosy. A higher frequency of Val/Val homozygosity occurred in leprosy patients as compared with controls (36% vs 5%; P < 0.001). Forty-two percent of MB and 17% of PB leprosy patients were positive for anti-beta2GPI IgM. SNPs Ser88Asn and Cys306Gly did not correlate with anti-beta2GPI antibody levels. MB patients with positive anti-beta2GPI IgM had higher frequency of Val/Val homozygosity than the controls (32% vs 15%; P = 0.042). The frequency of the mutant allele Ser316 was higher in MB patients with positive rather than negative anti-beta2GPI IgM levels (6% vs 0%; P = 0.040) and was greater than in the control group (6% vs 1%; P = 0.034). The studied polymorphisms did not influence the plasma concentrations of beta2GPI (Brochado et al., 2010).

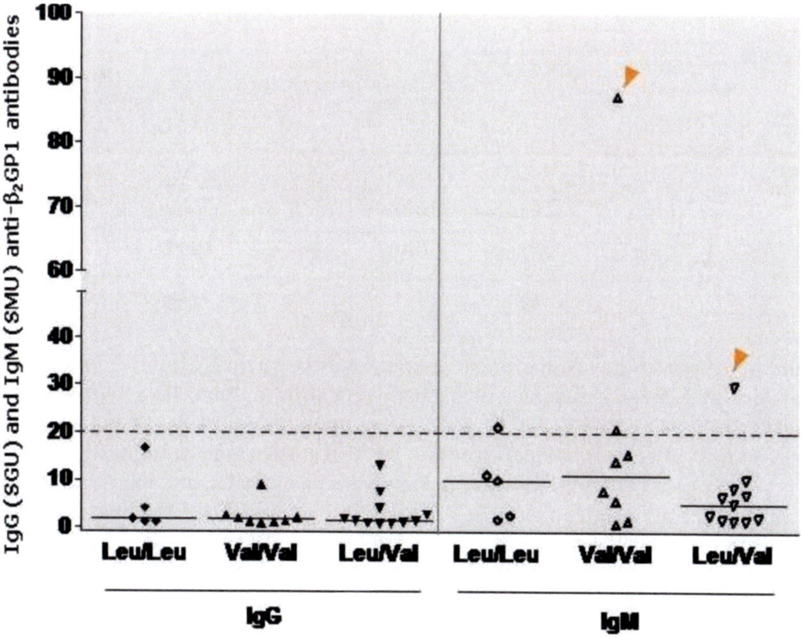

Figure 4A. Distribution of the titles of anti-β_2-glycoprotein 1 (β_2GP1) IgG and IgM antibodies by ELISA in samples of patients' sera with paucibacillary form of leprosy according to the Leu247Val *β_2GP1* gene polymorphisms. Horizontal line of each group: median. Stippled horizontal line: cut off = 20. The arrows indicate high titles of the IgM anti-β_2GP1 antibodies in PB leprosy, with the Leu/Val and Val/Val genotypes. Multiple Dunn's Test: $p > 0.05$ (Brochado et al., 2009).

Figure 4. (Continued)

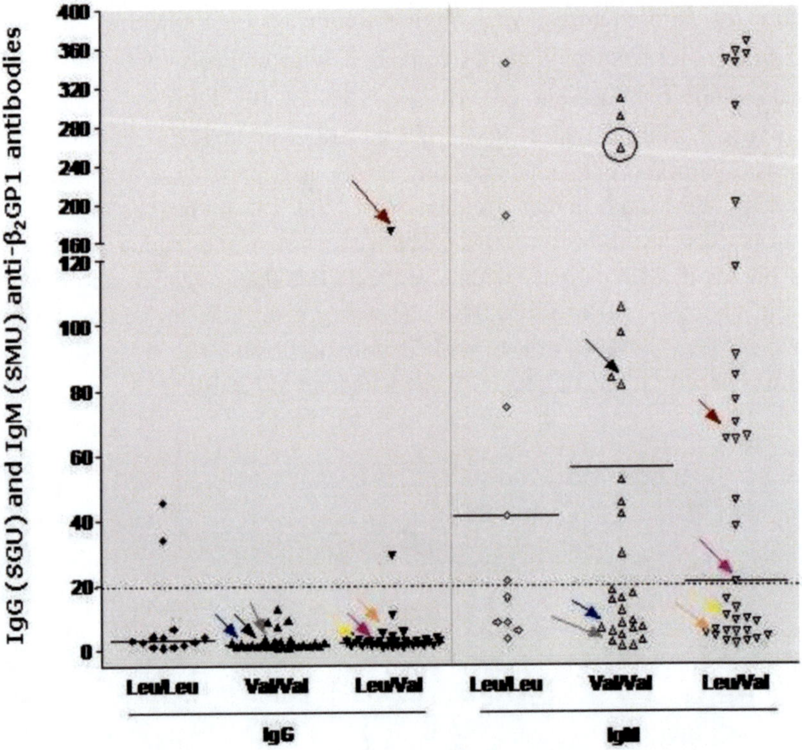

Figure 4B. Distribution of the titles of anti-β_2-glicoprotein 1 (β_2GP1) IgG and IgM antibodies by ELISA in samples of patients' sera with multibacillary form of leprosy according to the Leu247Val *β_2GP1* gene polymorphism. Horizontal line of each group: median. Stippled horizontal line: cut off = 20. The arrows indicate titles of anti-β_2GP1 antibodies in seven patients with thromboembolic phenomena, and the circle indicates the title in patient's sample that developed Lucio's phenomenon. Multiple Dunn's test: $p > 0.05$ (Brochado et al., 2009).

Our results attested that the Val/Val genotype prevailed in the leprosy group as compared with the controls. Regarding the seven MB patients with APS, four and three subjects presented heterozygosis and Val/Val homozygosis, respectively. Although higher titrations of anti-beta2GP1 IgM antibodies were seen in the PB and MB leprosy groups with the Leu/Val and Val/Val genotypes, no statistical difference existed as compared with the Leu/Leu genotype (Figures 4A and 4B).

In conclusion, our results suggest that Leu247Val and Trp316Ser SNPs may represent genetic risk factors for anti-β2GPI antibody production in MB leprosy patients. Hence, it is vital to improve the criteria for thalidomide prescription and anticoagulation therapy when antiphospholipid antibodies, such as anti-β2GPI, exist in MB leprosy patients, to avoid TEP and pulmonary embolization.

Instituting aPL signalization in the MB form of leprosy patients thus constitutes an improvement in the criteria for thalidomide prescription and anticoagulation therapy, to prevent TEP and pulmonary embolization.

References

Akerkar SM, Bichile LS. 2005. Leprosy & gangrene: a rare association; role of antiphospholipid antibodies. *BMC Infect. Dis*. 21;5:74.

Arvieux J, Renaudineau Y, Mane I, Perraut R, Krilis SA, Youinou P. 2002. Distinguishing features of anti-beta 2 glycoprotein I antibodies between patients with leprosy and the antiphospholipid syndrome. *Thromb. Haemost*. 87(4):599-605.

Atsumi T, Tsutsumi A, Amengual O, Khamashta MA, Hughes GR, Miyoshi Y, Ichikawa K, Koike T. 1999. Correlation between beta2-glycoprotein I valine/leucine247 polymorphism and anti-beta2-glycoprotein I antibodies in patients with primary antiphospholipid syndrome. *Rheumatology* (Oxford) 38:721–3.

Bakos L, Correa CC, Bergmann L, Bonamigo RR, Muller LF. 1996. Antiphospholipid antibodies thrombotic syndrome misdiagnosed as Lucio's phenomenon. *Int. J. Lepr. Other Mycobactb. Dis*. 64:320–3.

Brochado MJ, Figueiredo JF, Mendes-Junior CT, Louzada-Junior P, Kim OM, Roselino AM. 2010. Correlation between beta-2-glycoprotein I gene polymorphism and anti-beta-2 glycoprotein I antibodies in patients with multibacillary leprosy. *Arch. Dermatol. Res*. 302(8):583-91.

Brochado MJ, Nascimento MM, Louzada Junior P, Figueiredo JF, Roselino AM. 2009. Val247Leu polymorphism of beta2 glycoprotein 1 gene may justify the genesis of anti beta2GP1 antibodies and antiphospholipid syndrome in multibacillary leprosy. *An. Bras. Dermatol*. 84(4):355-9.

Cesarman-Maus G, Braggio E, Fonseca R. 2012. Thrombosis in multiple myeloma (MM). *Hematology*. 17 Suppl 1:S177-80.

Chen Q, Kamboh MI. 2006. Complete DNA sequence variation in the apolipoprotein H (beta-glycoprotein I) gene and identification of informative SNPs. *Ann. Hum. Genet.* 70:1–11.

de Larranaga GF, Forastiero RR, Martinuzzo ME, Carreras LO, Tsariktsian G, Sturno MM, Alonso BS. 2000. High prevalence of antiphospholipid antibodies in leprosy: evaluation of antigen reactivity. *Lupus.* 9:594–600.

Hebe Petiti-Martin G, Villar-Buill M, de la Hera I, Fuertes L, Burgués-Calderón M, Rivera-Díaz R, Vanaclocha F. 2013. Deep vein thrombosis in a patient with lepromatous leprosy receiving thalidomide to treat leprosy reaction. *Actas Dermosifiliogr.* 104(1):67-70.

Pierangeli SS, Vega-Ostertag ME, Gonzalez EB. 2007. New targeted therapies for treatment of thrombosis in antiphospholipid syndrome. *Expert Rev. Mol. Med.* 9(30):1-15.

Ribeiro SL, Pereira HL, Silva NP, Souza AW, Sato EI. 2011. Anti-β2-glycoprotein I antibodies are highly prevalent in a large number of Brazilian leprosy patients. *Acta Reumatol. Port.* 36(1):30-7.

Rogers JH. 1960. Coronary thrombosis, cerebral vascular accident and pulmonary embolism in leprosy. *Ann. Intern. Med.* 53:746-53.

Sène D, Piette JC, Cacoub P. 2008. Antiphospholipid antibodies, antiphospholipid syndrome and infections. *Autoimmun. Rev.* 7(4):272-7.

Sharma NL, Sharma V, Shanker V, Mahajan VK, Sarin S. 2004. Deep vein thrombosis: a rare complication of thalidomide therapy in recurrent erythema nodosum leprosum. *Int. J. Lepr. Other Mycobact. Dis.* 2004 Dec;72(4):483-5.

Vetrichevvel TP, Pise GA, Thappa DM. 2008. A case report of venous thrombosis in a leprosy patient treated with corticosteroid and thalidomide. *Lepr. Rev.* 79(2):193-5.

Yamaguchi S, Yamamoto Y, Hosokawa A, Hagiwara K, Uezato H, Takahashi K. 2012. Deep venous thrombosis and pulmonary embolism secondary to co-administration of thalidomide and oral corticosteroid in a patient with leprosy. *J. Dermatol.* 39(8):711-4.

Genetic Markers on Leprosy

Leprosy, caused by the obligate intracellular microorganism *M. leprae*, is a chronic disabling disease that remains a major health problem in some African, Asian and Latin American countries (WHO 2012).

It is characterized by a spectrum of clinical manifestations—from tuberculoid to lepromatous poles—that correlate with host cell-mediated immunity against the bacillus. Besides environmental and lifestyle factors, host genetic susceptibility has been attributed to the clinical diversity of the disease. Recent studies on both innate and adaptive immune responses to *M. leprae* have provided hypotheses for candidate gene association studies.

Because a comprehensive report of such genetic polymorphisms in a Brazilian leprosy sample is not available, we have investigated the association between the polymorphisms of the solute carrier family 11 member 1 gene (*SLC11A1*), also known as *NRAMP1* (natural resistance-associated macrophage protein 1), and the polymorphisms of the genes related with inflammation, susceptibility, or resistance to leprosy.

Association of the Solute Carrier Family 11 Member 1 Gene (*SLC11A1/NRAMP1*) polymorphisms with Susceptibility to Leprosy

The solute carrier family 11 member 1 gene (*SLC11A1*), also known as *NRAMP1* (natural resistance-associated macrophage protein 1), is a gene that controls the susceptibility of inbred mice to intracellular pathogens, including *Mycobacterium*, *Salmonella*, and *Leishmania* microorganisms (Vidal et al., 1993).

Susceptibility to infection in inbred laboratory mice originates from a single nonconservative glycine-to-aspartic acid substitution at position 169 within the transmembrane domain 4 of *SLC11A1/NRAMP1* (Malo et al., 1994; Vidal et al., 1996). The human homologue *SLC11A1/NRAMP1* has been cloned, and several variants within the *SLC11A1/NRAMP1* gene have been described, but the functional significance of these variants remains uncertain (Cellier et al., 1994; Liu et al., 1995). Functionally, murine NRAMP proteins influence pathogen viability and/or replication within macrophages by transporting iron and other divalent cations across the phagosomal membrane (Gruenheid and Gros, 2000).

Several reports have shown that the *NRAMP1/SLC11A1* polymorphisms are associated with host susceptibility to tuberculosis and leprosy (Abel et al., 1998; Meisner et al., 2001; Hatta et al., 2010; Li et al., 2011). In this regard, a population-based association study in Brazil demonstrated that lepromin-negative individuals harboring specific genotypes of a (GT)n promoter repeat of *SLC11A1/NRAMP1* were at risk of developing leprosy, which suggested an interaction between genetic and immunological factors (Ferreira et al., 2004).

In our case-control study, we evaluated nine polymorphisms [(GT)n, 274C/T, 469+14G/C, 577-18G/A, 823C/T, A318V, 1465-85G/A, D543N, and 1729+55del4] of the *NRAMP1/SLC11A1* gene in 86 leprosy outpatients affiliated with the University Hospital of the School of Medicine of Ribeirao Preto (HC-FMRP), University of Sao Paulo (USP). Among these participants, 67 patients were classified as having multibacillary (MB) leprosy including the mid-borderline (BB), borderline tuberculoid (BT), borderline lepromatous (BL), and Lepromatous Leprosy (LL) clinical forms.

The other 19 patients were classified as paucibacillary (PB) leprosy, including the TT and BT clinical forms, following Ridley and Jopling classification. Criteria for classification of PB leprosy included lack of bacilli in lymph smears, skin biopsies, or nerve biopsies and ≤5 skin lesions.

The control group consisted of 239 blood donors affiliated with the Hemocentro Blood Bank (HC-FMRP, USP) from the same region, matched for age, gender, and skin color. None of these individuals showed any evidence of previous underlying diseases; they were also serologically negative for Chagas' disease, hepatitis B and C, and HIV infection.

PCR followed by enzymatic restriction aided detection of the *SLC11A1/NRAMP1* gene polymorphisms (Liu et al., 1995).

From a statistical viewpoint, the leprosy and control groups did not differ in terms of the genotypic and allelic frequencies of the *SLC11A1/NRAMP1* 577-18G/A, 823C/T, A318V, 1465-85G/A, D543N, and 1729+55del4 polymorphisms.

Regarding the (GT)n polymorphism, the frequency of allele 2 in leprosy patients was higher than in the control group (32% vs 24%, P = 0.04; OR = 1.49, 95% CI = 1.02-2.18), whereas the frequency of allele 3 was higher in the control group (74% vs 65%, P = 0.03; OR = 0.66, 95% CI = 0.45-0.96).

Analysis of the 274C/T polymorphism revealed increased frequency of the 274T allele (33% vs 24%, P = 0.04; OR = 1.49, 95% CI = 1.02-2.18) and the T/T genotype (14% vs 7%, P = 0.02; OR = 2.46, 95% CI = 1.08-5.62) among leprosy patients as compared with the control group.

Similarly, a significantly higher frequency of the 469+14C allele of the 469+14G/C polymorphism occurred in leprosy patients (30% vs 23%, P = 0.03; OR = 1.53, 95% CI = 1.03-2.25). None of the nine polymorphisms of the *SLC11A1/NRAMP1* gene were significantly different among the leprosy subgroups (Table 1). The genotype distributions in the control group agreed with the Hardy–Weinberg equilibrium (HWE) for all the polymorphisms.

Briefly, our results demonstrated that the polymorphisms 274C/T in exon 3 and 469+14G/C in intron 4 of the *SLC11A1/NRAMP1* gene were associated with susceptibility to leprosy.

The (GT)n polymorphisms in the promoter region of the *SLC11A1/NRAMP1* gene were associated with protection against or susceptibility to leprosy.

Positive and negative associations between leprosy and the *NRAMP1/SLC11A1* gene polymorphisms have been described (Roy et al., 1999; Fitness et al., 2004; Hatta et al., 2010). Hatta et al. (2010) evaluated three variants of the *NRAMP1/SLC11A1* gene (D543N, 1929+55del4 and 469+14G/C) in leprosy patients from Indonesia and found an association of the 469+14GC genotype of the 469+14G/C polymorphism among leprosy per se and PB leprosy.

In case control studies conducted in Mali, the 3'untranslated region (3' UTR) (1729+55del4) polymorphism was associated with MB leprosy but not with leprosy per se (Meisner et al., 2001). However, candidate gene studies in a population from northern Malawi (Fitness et al., 2004), India (Roy et al., 1999), and Thailand (Vejbaesya et al., 2007) failed to detect any association between *NRAMP1/SLC11A1* polymorphisms and leprosy.

In our study, we observed that the frequency of the allele 2 (GT)n polymorphism in the promoter region of the *SLC11A1/NRAMP1* gene was higher in the leprosy group, which suggested association with susceptibility to leprosy. Similarly to our results, Ferreira et al. (2004) observed that individuals with a negative lepromin response associated with genotypes 22 and 23 presented greater risk of developing leprosy.

Discrepancies exist in the polymorphisms of *SLC11A1/NRAMP1* associated with the disease, and the functional significance of the polymorphisms remains unclear. In the mouse model, the *SLC11A1/NRAMP1* alleles influence the intrinsic ability of macrophages to resist infection by intracellular parasites (Skamene, 1994).

Other studies have shown that the *SLC11A1/NRAMP1* locus encodes a protein that also exerts pleiotropic effects including regulation of the T helper 1 (Th1) / T helper 2 (Th2) balance of the adaptive immune response to infection (Soo et al., 1998; Blackwell et al., 2000). It is very important to identify the genetic factors that regulate the Th1/Th2 balance in response to foreign antigens.

The polymorphisms of the *SLC11A1/NRAMP1* gene could play an important role in the immune response type in leprosy.

Table 1. Allelic and genotypic frequencies of the *SLC11A1/NRAMP1* polymorphisms in the leprosy and control groups

Polymorphism site	Alleles/ Genotypes	Leprosy (n = 86)	MB (n = 67)	PB (n = 19)	Controls (n = 239)
Promoter microsatellite (GT)n repeat	Alleles [n, (%)]				
	1	1 (0.5)	1 (0.5)	0(0)	4 (1)
	2	56 (32.5)	43 (32)	13 (34)	117 (24)*
	3	112 (65)	88 (66)	24 (63)	353 (74)**
	5	3 (2)	2 (1.5)	1 (3)	4 (1)
	Genotype [n, (%)]				
	12	0 (0)	0 (0)	0 (0)	1 (0.5)
	13	1 (1)	1 (1.5)	0 (0)	3 (1)
	22	13 (15)	11 (16.5)	2 (11)	16 (7)
	23	28 (33)	20 (30)	8 (42)	83 (35)
	25	2 (2)	1 (1.5)	1 (5)	1 (0.5)
	33	41 (48)	33 (49)	8 (42)	132 (55)
	35	1 (1)	1 (1.5)	0 (0)	3 (1)
Exon 3 274 C/T	Alleles [n, (%)]				
	C	116 (67)	92 (68)	24 (63)	361 (76)
	T	56 (33)	42 (32)	14 (37)	117 (24)§
	Genotype [n, (%)]				
	CC	42 (49)	34 (51)	8 (42)	138 (58)
	CT	32 (37)	24 (36)	8 (42)	85 (35)
	TT	12 (14)	9 (13)	3 (16)	16 (7)§ §
Intron 4 469+14 G/C	Alleles [n, (%)]				
	C	53 (30)	40 (30)	13 (34)	108 (23) †
	G	119 (70)	94 (70)	25 (66)	370 (77)
	Genotype [n, (%)]				
	CC	10 (12)	8 (12)	2 (11)	14 (6)
	CG	33 (38)	24 (36)	9 (47)	80 (33)
	GG	43 (50)	35 (52)	8 (42)	145 (61)

(GT)n polymorphism: * Allele 2 [P = 0.04; OR = 1.49, 95% CI = 1.02-2.18] /**Allele 3 [P = 0.03; OR = 0.66, 95% CI = 0.45-0.96].

274C/T polymorphism: § 274T allele [P = 0.04; OR = 1.49, 95% CI = 1.02-2.18] / § § TT genotype [P = 0.02; OR = 2.46, 95%CI = 1.08-5.62].

469+14G/C polymorphism: † 469+14C allele [P = 0.03; OR = 1.53, 95% CI = 1.03-2.25].

References

Abel, L., Sanchez, F. O., Oberti, J., Thuc, N. V., Hoa, L. V., Lap, V. D., Skamene, E., Lagrange, P. H. and Schurr, E., 1998. Susceptibility to leprosy is linked to the human NRAMP1 gene. *J. Infect. Dis.* 177, 133-45.

Blackwell, J. M., Searle, S., Goswami, T. and Miller, E. N., 2000. Understanding the multiple functions of Nramp1. *Microbes Infect.* 2, 317-21.

Cellier, M., Govoni, G., Vidal, S., Kwan, T., Groulx, N., Liu, J., Sanchez, F., Skamene, E., Schurr, E. and Gros, P., 1994. Human natural resistance-associated macrophage protein: cDNA cloning, chromosomal mapping, genomic organization, and tissue-specific expression. *J. Exp. Med.* 180, 1741-52.

Ferreira, F. R., Goulart, L. R., Silva, H. D. and Goulart, I. M., 2004. Susceptibility to leprosy may be conditioned by an interaction between the NRAMP1 promoter polymorphisms and the lepromin response. *Int. J. Lepr. Other Mycobact. Dis.* 72, 457-67.

Fitness, J., Floyd, S., Warndorff, D. K., Sichali, L., Mwaungulu, L., Crampin, A. C., Fine, P. E. and Hill, A. V., 2004. Large-scale candidate gene study of leprosy susceptibility in the Karonga district of northern Malawi. *Am. J. Trop. Med. Hyg.* 71, 330-40.

Gruenheid, S. and Gros, P., 2000. Genetic susceptibility to intracellular infections: Nramp1, macrophage function and divalent cations transport. *Curr. Opin. Microbiol.* 3, 43-8.

Hatta, M., Ratnawati, Tanaka, M., Ito, J., Shirakawa, T. and Kawabata, M., 2010. NRAMP1/SLC11A1 gene polymorphisms and host susceptibility to Mycobacterium tuberculosis and M. leprae in South Sulawesi, Indonesia. *Southeast Asian J. Trop. Med. Public Health* 41, 386-94.

Li, X., Yang, Y., Zhou, F., Zhang, Y., Lu, H., Jin, Q. and Gao, L., 2011. SLC11A1 (NRAMP1) polymorphisms and tuberculosis susceptibility: updated systematic review and meta-analysis. *PLoS One* 6, e15831.

Liu, J., Fujiwara, T.M., Buu, N.T., Sanchez, F.O., Cellier, M., Paradis, A.J., Frappier, D., Skamene, E., Gros, P., Morgan, K. and et al., 1995. Identification of polymorphisms and sequence variants in the human homologue of the mouse natural resistance-associated macrophage protein gene. *Am. J. Hum. Genet.* 56, 845-53.

Malo, D., Vogan, K., Vidal, S., Hu, J., Cellier, M., Schurr, E., Fuks, A., Bumstead, N., Morgan, K. and Gros, P., 1994. Haplotype mapping and sequence analysis of the mouse Nramp gene predict susceptibility to infection with intracellular parasites. *Genomics* 23, 51-61.

Meisner, S.J., Mucklow, S., Warner, G., Sow, S.O., Lienhardt, C. and Hill, A.V., 2001. Association of NRAMP1 polymorphism with leprosy type but not susceptibility to leprosy per se in west Africans. *Am. J. Trop. Med. Hyg.* 65, 733-5.

Roy, S., Frodsham, A., Saha, B., Hazra, S.K., Mascie-Taylor, C.G. and Hill, A.V., 1999. Association of vitamin D receptor genotype with leprosy type. *J. Infect. Dis.* 179, 187-91.

Skamene, E., 1994. The Bcg gene story. *Immunobiology* 191, 451-60.

Soo, S. S., Villarreal-Ramos, B., Anjam Khan, C. M., Hormaeche, C. E. and Blackwell, J. M., 1998. Genetic control of immune response to recombinant antigens carried by an attenuated Salmonella typhimurium vaccine strain: Nramp1 influences T-helper subset responses and protection against leishmanial challenge. *Infect. Immun.* 66, 1910-7.

Vejbaesya, S., Mahaisavariya, P., Luangtrakool, P. and Sermduangprateep, C., 2007. TNF alpha and NRAMP1 polymorphisms in leprosy. *J. Med. Assoc. Thai* 90, 1188-92.

Vidal, S. M., Malo, D., Vogan, K., Skamene, E. and Gros, P., 1993. Natural resistance to infection with intracellular parasites: isolation of a candidate for Bcg. *Cell* 73, 469-85.

Vidal, S. M., Pinner, E., Lepage, P., Gauthier, S. and Gros, P., 1996. Natural resistance to intracellular infections: Nramp1 encodes a membrane phosphoglycoprotein absent in macrophages from susceptible (Nramp1 D169) mouse strains. *J. Immunol.* 157, 3559-68.

WHO (2012). "Global leprosy situation, 2012." Weekly epidemiological record 87 317–328: 317–328.

Genetic Polymorphisms of Innate and Adaptive Immune Response and Susceptibility to Leprosy

Leprosy is characterized by clinically defined polar manifestations that depend upon the host cell–mediated immune response against the pathogen. The tuberculoid (TT) and lepromatous (LL) poles of leprosy are associated with either a strong cell-mediated immunity and T helper 1 (Th1) cytokine profile or a T helper 2 (Th2) cytokine profile and strong humoral response, respectively (Scollard et al., 2006a). The intermediate clinical forms, termed borderline (BT, BB, BL), are classified according to their proximity to each pole (Ridley and Jopling, 1966).

Throughout the natural course of the disease, patients can also develop clinical complications such as the leprosy reactions (LR). LR consist of intense and sudden activation/reactivation of the host immune/inflammatory responses that frequently affect the peripheral nerves (Fava et al., 2012). Two major types of LR exist: type-1 reaction (T1R) or reversal reaction, and type-2 reaction (T2R) or erythema nodosum leprosum. Although they are clinically different, both types can lead to severe nerve damage and disabilities (Kahawita and Lockwood, 2008; Walker and Lockwood, 2008).

Several research lines, including twin studies, genome-wide linkage studies, candidate gene association studies, and genome-wide association studies (GWAS), have indicated that host genetic factors help to determine susceptibility to *Mycobacteria* (Misch et al., 2010). Recent studies of the innate and adaptive immune responses to *M. leprae* have provided hypotheses for candidate gene association studies (Cardoso et al., 2011).

Genetic studies on the receptors that mediate *Mycobacteria* recognition, including toll-like receptors (*TLR4*) (Bochud et al., 2009), vitamin D receptor (*VDR*) (Roy et al., 1999), and the mannose binding lectins (*MBL*) (Sapkota et al., 2010), have shown association between leprosy phenotypes and polymorphisms.

Polymorphic variants located on different functional promoter regions for cytokine genes, such as tumor necrosis factor-alpha (*TNF-α*) (Santos et al., 2002), lymphotoxin-alpha (*LTA*) (Alcais et al., 2007), interleukin (IL)-10 (*IL-10*) (Santos et al., 2002), *IL-6*, and IL-1 receptor antagonist (*IL-1Ra*) (Settin et al., 2007) have also been associated with susceptibility to or protection against leprosy as well as the clinical outcome of this disease.

While a significant number of reports have described some polymorphic genes in different leprosy populations, the literature does not contain a comprehensive study of such genetic polymorphisms in a Brazilian leprosy sample.

Here, we investigated associations of the polymorphisms in innate immune receptors (*TLR4* 896A/G; *VDR Bsm*I, *VDR Apa*I and *VDR Taq*I) and cytokines (*TNF-α* -308G/A; *IL-10* -1082G/A, *IL-6* -174G/C, and *IL-1Ra* 86bp VNTR) genes with susceptibility/resistance to leprosy and leprosy clinical forms.

This study involved a total of 86 leprosy patients [67 multibacillary (MB) and 19 paucibacillary (PB) forms of leprosy] and 239 healthy controls matched for age, sex, and ethnicity to the patients, as described previously.

Polymerase chain reaction-restriction fragment length polymorphism protocols (PCR-RFLP) or RT-qPCR with TaqMan probes aided genotyping for each gene variation, conducted according to previously published methods (Wilson et al., 1992; Tarlow et al., 1993; Turner et al., 1997; Fishman et al., 1998; Pieroni et al., 2007).

The present study revealed that the leprosy patients and control group were similar in terms of the genotypic and allelic frequencies of *TLR4* 896A/G*; VDR Bsm*I, *VDR Apa*I, and *VDR Taq*I; and *IL-6* -174G/C, and *IL-1Ra* 86bp VNTR.

However, significantly higher frequency of the AA genotype of the *TNF-α* -308G/A polymorphism existed in the total leprosy group (6%) and in the MB group (7%) as compared with the control group (1%) ($P = 0.04$; OR = 4.7, 95% CI = 1.1-20.8 and $P = 0.03$; OR = 6.2, 95% CI = 1.4-27.0; respectively). Analysis of the -1082G/A polymorphism in the *IL-10* promoter region showed increased frequency of the -1082A allele (79% vs 62%, $P = 0.03$; OR = 2.31, 95% CI = 1.03-5.14) and the AA genotype (63% vs 39%, $P = 0.04$; OR = 2.69, 95% CI = 1.02-7.08) among PB patients as compared with the control group (Table 2). The genotype frequencies did not deviate significantly from HWE for the controls.

Our main findings were the association of (i) the *TNF-α* -308G/A polymorphism with susceptibility to leprosy per se and MB leprosy, and (ii) the *IL-10* -1082G/A polymorphism with susceptibility to the PB form of the disease. These polymorphisms will be briefly discussed here.

TNF-α is a multifunctional proinflammatory cytokine produced by monocytes and macrophages. It plays a major role in nonspecific inflammation and innate resistance and constitutes one of the most powerful stimulants of cell-mediated immunity (Scollard et al., 2006a). TNF-α is especially important in leprosy: it stabilizes granuloma formation and is implicated in the pathophysiology of the reactional states of leprosy (Sarno et al., 1991; Moraes et al., 1999; Scollard et al., 2006b).

The *TNF-α* gene cluster is located within the class III region of the highly polymorphic major histocompatibility complex (MHC) on human chromosome 6p21. Several polymorphisms in the promoter region of the *TNF-α* gene have been identified (Hajeer and Hutchinson, 2001). Bearing in mind that the range of TNF-α effects on cellular immunity is wide, these promoter polymorphisms are extremely interesting—they might modulate the degree of host response and therefore the clinical types of leprosy (Scollard et al., 2006a). Several genetic studies have reported associations of the *TNF-α* -308G/A polymorphism with susceptibility to or protection against leprosy

(Roy et al., 1997; Santos et al., 2002; Vejbaesya et al., 2007; Franceschi et al., 2009).

The association of the *TNF-α* -308A allele with susceptibility to leprosy observed in the present study confirmed the results of several previous investigations (Roy et al., 1997; Vejbaesya et al., 2007). Roy et al. (Roy et al., 1997) were the first to verify this association; they also observed that the frequency of the TNF -308A allele was higher in LL patients as compared with healthy individuals. Vejbaesya et al. (Vejbaesya et al., 2007) reported similar findings for leprosy patients from Thailand. They showed association of this polymorphism with susceptibility to the MB form of leprosy. Studies from southern Brazil (Santos et al., 2002) and Nepal (Sapkota et al., 2010) reported the opposite result: they verified that the *TNF-α* -308A allele was associated with protection against leprosy as compared with healthy controls. In contrast to the studies mentioned above, Fitness et al. (Fitness et al., 2004) and Felix et al. (Velarde Felix et al., 2012) did not find association of this polymorphism with susceptibility to leprosy in patients from Northern Malawi and Northwest Mexico, respectively. These contradictory results may have stemmed from ethnic differences among the study populations or the natural history of leprosy in diverse geographic settings. Even though the exact nature of the association remains controversial, these studies suggest that the *TNF-α* gene participates in a complex mechanism of genetic control of susceptibility or resistance to leprosy (Mira, 2006).

IL-10 is a potent anti-inflammatory and immunosuppressive cytokine that regulates protective immunity in leprosy. IL-10 is enhanced in the MB form of the disease (Misra et al., 1995), and a higher TNF-*α* /IL-10 ratio is correlated with better prognosis in terms of clinical outcome of leprosy in household contacts (Lima et al., 2000). The *IL-10* polymorphisms in the distal and the proximal regions are arranged to form haplotypes in the promoter gene; these combinations have been associated with secretion of the cytokine *in vitro* (Yilmaz et al., 2005).

Genetic variants of the *IL-10* promoter gene, such as -1082G/A, -819C/T, and -592C/A, alone or in haplotype, have been studied; however, discordant results have been noted (Santos et al., 2002; Malhotra et al., 2005; Franceschi et al., 2009; Cardona-Castro et al., 2012). Our present data demonstrate that, in our population, the genotype *IL-10* -1082AA and the allele *IL-10* -1082A were associated with the susceptibility to the PB form of the disease. In contrast to our results, several genetic studies have not found any association of this polymorphism with leprosy (Fitness et al., 2004; Moraes et al., 2004; Cardona-Castro et al., 2012).

Table 2. Allelic and genotypic frequencies of the cytokines polymorphisms in leprosy and control groups

Gene / Polymorphism site	Alleles/ Genotypes	MB (n = 67)	PB (n = 19)	All Leprosy (n = 86)	Controls (n = 239)	*P*-value	OR (95% IC)
Tumor necrosis factor-alpha							
Promoter region	Alleles [n, (%)]						
(-308 G→A)	G	112 (84)	36 (95)	148 (86)	424 (89)		
	A	22 (16)	2 (5)	24 (14)	54 (11)		
	Genotype [n, (%)]						
	AA	5 (7)	0 (0)	5 (6)	3 (1)	0.05	4.7 (1.1 - 20.1)†
	GA	12 (18)	2 (11)	14 (16)	48 (20)	0.03	4.9 (1.1 - 20.8)‡
	GG	50 (75)	17(89)	67 (78)	188 (79)	0.03	6.26 (1.4 - 27.0)*
						0.01	6.34 (1.4 - 27.2)**
Interleukin-10	Alleles [n, (%)]						
Promoter region	G	49 (36)	8 (21)	57 (33)	182 (38)	0.03	2.31 (1.03-5.14)§
(−1082 G→A)	A	85 (64)	30 (79)	115 (67)	296 (62)		
	Genotype [n, (%)]						
	GG	9 (14)	1 (5)	10 (12)	36 (15)		
	GA	31 (46)	6 (32)	37 (43)	110 (46)		
	AA	27 (40)	12 (63)	39 (45)	93 (39)	0.04	2.69 (1.02 - 7.08) §§

† Leprosy vs controls [AA vs GG] / ‡ Leprosy vs controls [AA vs GA+GG] / * Multibacillary (MB) vs controls [AA vs GG] / ** MB vs controls [AA vs GA+GG] / § Paucibacillary (PB) vs Controls / §§ PB vs Controls [AA vs GA+GG]

In a study in Egypt, the genotype *IL-10* -1082GG was associated with susceptibility to leprosy per se and PB leprosy (Settin et al., 2007). The involvement of different *IL-10* genotypes, alleles, and haplotypes in the outcome of leprosy in different ethnic populations suggests that it is necessary to investigate the *IL-10* region further by means of both genetic and functional studies.

Conclusion

Since the *M. leprae* bacillus is not yet cultivable, newer tests are necessary to detect this microorganism mainly in patients with the PB form of leprosy and in people who were in contact with the patient. Here, primers that can sensitively (up to 85% sensitivity) and specifically (100% specificity) detect the Ml *MntH* (ML2098) gene of the *M. leprae* by PCR and qPCR have been developed and successfully employed in several examined human samples.

Increased values of anti-beta2GP1 IgM antibodies occur in the MB form of leprosy associated with the Leu247Val and Trp316Ser polymorphisms of the *Beta2GP1* gene, justifying a genetic risk factor for antiphospholipid antibody syndrome and the TEP detected in seven leprosy patients. Therefore, the criteria used to prescribe thalidomide and anticoagulation therapy must be improved when antiphospholipid antibodies, such as anti-β2GPI, exist in MB leprosy patients, to avoid TEP and pulmonary embolization.

Regarding genetic studies on leprosy, our results demonstrated that the polymorphisms 274C/T in exon 3 and 469+14G/C in intron 4 of the *SLC11A1/NRAMP1* gene were associated with susceptibility to leprosy. The (GT)n polymorphisms in the promoter region of the *SLC11A1/NRAMP1* gene were associated with protection against or susceptibility to leprosy. Genetic polymorphisms related to *TNF-α* -308G/A and *IL-10* -1082G/A might constitute genetic markers for susceptibility to and clinical outcome of leprosy.

Given the current challenge in eliminating leprosy, especially in remaining endemic countries, we hope our studies will contribute to new perspectives for treatment and prevention of the disease.

Acknowledgments

We are very thankful for the technical assistance of Maria Fernanda Chociay-Gatti, Ph.D. We also thank Professor Marco Antonio Zago, M.D., Ph.D., for offering the laboratory for the inflammatory genetic study.

These studies were supported by CNPq, FAPESP, and FAEPA.

References

Alcais, A., Alter, A., Antoni, G., Orlova, M., Nguyen, V. T., Singh, M., Vanderborght, P. R., Katoch, K., Mira, M. T., Vu, H. T., Ngyuen, T. H., Nguyen, N. B., Moraes, M., Mehra, N., Schurr, E. and Abel, L., 2007. Stepwise replication identifies a low-producing lymphotoxin-alpha allele as a major risk factor for early-onset leprosy. *Nat. Genet.* 39, 517-22.

Bochud, P. Y., Sinsimer, D., Aderem, A., Siddiqui, M. R., Saunderson, P., Britton, S., Abraham, I., Tadesse Argaw, A., Janer, M., Hawn, T. R. and Kaplan, G., 2009. Polymorphisms in Toll-like receptor 4 (TLR4) are associated with protection against leprosy. *Eur. J. Clin. Microbiol. Infect. Dis.* 28, 1055-65.

Cardona-Castro, N., Sanchez-Jimenez, M., Rojas, W. and Bedoya-Berrio, G., 2012. IL-10 gene promoter polymorphisms and leprosy in a Colombian population sample. *Biomedica* 32, 71-6.

Cardoso, C. C., Pereira, A. C., de Sales Marques, C. and Moraes, M. O., 2011. Leprosy susceptibility: genetic variations regulate innate and adaptive immunity, and disease outcome. *Future Microbiol.* 6, 533-49.

Fava, V., Orlova, M., Cobat, A., Alcais, A., Mira, M. and Schurr, E., 2012. Genetics of leprosy reactions: an overview. *Mem. Inst. Oswaldo Cruz* 107 Suppl 1, 132-42.

Fishman, D., Faulds, G., Jeffery, R., Mohamed-Ali, V., Yudkin, J. S., Humphries, S. and Woo, P., 1998. The effect of novel polymorphisms in the interleukin-6 (IL-6) gene on IL-6 transcription and plasma IL-6 levels, and an association with systemic-onset juvenile chronic arthritis. *J. Clin. Invest.* 102, 1369-76.

Fitness, J., Floyd, S., Warndorff, D. K., Sichali, L., Mwaungulu, L., Crampin, A. C., Fine, P. E. and Hill, A. V., 2004. Large-scale candidate gene study of leprosy susceptibility in the Karonga district of northern Malawi. *Am. J. Trop. Med. Hyg.* 71, 330-40.

Franceschi, D. S., Mazini, P. S., Rudnick, C. C., Sell, A. M., Tsuneto, L. T., Ribas, M. L., Peixoto, P. R. and Visentainer, J. E., 2009. Influence of TNF and IL10 gene polymorphisms in the immunopathogenesis of leprosy in the south of Brazil. *Int. J. Infect. Dis*. 13, 493-8.

Hajeer, A. H. and Hutchinson, I. V., 2001. Influence of TNFalpha gene polymorphisms on TNFalpha production and disease. *Hum. Immunol*. 62, 1191-9.

Kahawita, I. P. and Lockwood, D. N., 2008. Towards understanding the pathology of erythema nodosum leprosum. *Trans. R. Soc. Trop. Med. Hyg*. 102, 329-37.

Lima, M. C., Pereira, G. M., Rumjanek, F. D., Gomes, H. M., Duppre, N., Sampaio, E. P., Alvim, I. M., Nery, J. A., Sarno, E. N. and Pessolani, M. C., 2000. Immunological cytokine correlates of protective immunity and pathogenesis in leprosy. *Scand. J. Immunol*. 51, 419-28.

Malhotra, D., Darvishi, K., Sood, S., Sharma, S., Grover, C., Relhan, V., Reddy, B. S. and Bamezai, R. N., 2005. IL-10 promoter single nucleotide polymorphisms are significantly associated with resistance to leprosy. *Hum. Genet*. 118, 295-300.

Mira, M. T., 2006. Genetic host resistance and susceptibility to leprosy. *Microbes Infect*. 8, 1124-31.

Misch, E. A., Berrington, W. R., Vary, J. C., Jr. and Hawn, T. R., 2010. Leprosy and the human genome. *Microbiol. Mol. Biol. Rev*. 74, 589-620.

Misra, N., Murtaza, A., Walker, B., Narayan, N. P., Misra, R. S., Ramesh, V., Singh, S., Colston, M. J. and Nath, I., 1995. Cytokine profile of circulating T cells of leprosy patients reflects both indiscriminate and polarized T-helper subsets: T-helper phenotype is stable and uninfluenced by related antigens of Mycobacterium leprae. *Immunology* 86, 97-103.

Moraes, M. O., Pacheco, A. G., Schonkeren, J. J., Vanderborght, P. R., Nery, J. A., Santos, A. R., Moraes, M. E., Moraes, J. R., Ottenhoff, T. H., Sampaio, E. P., Huizinga, T. W. and Sarno, E. N., 2004. Interleukin-10 promoter single-nucleotide polymorphisms as markers for disease susceptibility and disease severity in leprosy. *Genes Immun*. 5, 592-5.

Moraes, M. O., Sarno, E. N., Almeida, A. S., Saraiva, B. C., Nery, J. A., Martins, R. C. and Sampaio, E. P., 1999. Cytokine mRNA expression in leprosy: a possible role for interferon-gamma and interleukin-12 in reactions (RR and ENL). *Scand. J. Immunol*. 50, 541-9.

Pieroni, F., Lourenco, D. M., Morelli, V. M., Maffei, F. H., Zago, M. A. and Franco, R. F., 2007. Cytokine gene variants and venous thrombotic risk in the BRATROS (*Brazilian Thrombosis Study*). *Thromb. Res*. 120, 221-9.

Ridley, D. S. and Jopling, W. H., 1966. Classification of leprosy according to immunity. A five-group system. *Int. J. Lepr. Other Mycobact. Dis.* 34, 255-73.

Roy, S., Frodsham, A., Saha, B., Hazra, S. K., Mascie-Taylor, C. G. and Hill, A. V., 1999. Association of vitamin D receptor genotype with leprosy type. *J. Infect. Dis.* 179, 187-91.

Roy, S., McGuire, W., Mascie-Taylor, C. G., Saha, B., Hazra, S. K., Hill, A. V. and Kwiatkowski, D., 1997. Tumor necrosis factor promoter polymorphism and susceptibility to lepromatous leprosy. *J. Infect. Dis.* 176, 530-2.

Santos, A. R., Suffys, P. N., Vanderborght, P. R., Moraes, M. O., Vieira, L. M., Cabello, P. H., Bakker, A. M., Matos, H. J., Huizinga, T. W., Ottenhoff, T. H., Sampaio, E. P. and Sarno, E. N., 2002. Role of tumor necrosis factor-alpha and interleukin-10 promoter gene polymorphisms in leprosy. *J. Infect. Dis.* 186, 1687-91.

Sapkota, B. R., Macdonald, M., Berrington, W. R., Misch, E. A., Ranjit, C., Siddiqui, M. R., Kaplan, G. and Hawn, T. R., 2010. Association of TNF, MBL, and VDR polymorphisms with leprosy phenotypes. *Hum. Immunol.* 71, 992-8.

Sarno, E. N., Grau, G. E., Vieira, L. M. and Nery, J. A., 1991. Serum levels of tumour necrosis factor-alpha and interleukin-1 beta during leprosy reactional states. *Clin. Exp. Immunol.* 84, 103-8.

Scollard, D. M., Adams, L. B., Gillis, T. P., Krahenbuhl, J. L., Truman, R. W. and Williams, D. L., 2006a. The continuing challenges of leprosy. *Clin. Microbiol. Rev.* 19, 338-81.

Scollard, D. M., Joyce, M. P. and Gillis, T. P., 2006b. Development of leprosy and type 1 leprosy reactions after treatment with infliximab: a report of 2 cases. *Clin. Infect. Dis.* 43, e19-22.

Settin, A., Nassar, S., Abdel-Latif, A., Elbaz, R., El-Mongy, S. and Hassan, A., 2007. Association of cytokine gene polymorphism with susceptibility and clinical types of leprosy. *Int. J. Health Sci.* (Qassim) 1, 25-33.

Tarlow, J. K., Blakemore, A. I., Lennard, A., Solari, R., Hughes, H. N., Steinkasserer, A. and Duff, G. W., 1993. Polymorphism in human IL-1 receptor antagonist gene intron 2 is caused by variable numbers of an 86-bp tandem repeat. *Hum. Genet.* 91, 403-4.

Turner, D. M., Williams, D. M., Sankaran, D., Lazarus, M., Sinnott, P. J. and Hutchinson, I. V., 1997. An investigation of polymorphism in the interleukin-10 gene promoter. *Eur. J. Immunogenet.* 24, 1-8.

Vejbaesya, S., Mahaisavariya, P., Luangtrakool, P. and Sermduangprateep, C., 2007. TNF alpha and NRAMP1 polymorphisms in leprosy. *J. Med. Assoc. Thai* 90, 1188-92.

Velarde Felix, J. S., Cazarez-Salazar, S., Rios-Tostado, J. J., Flores-Garcia, A., Rangel-Villalobos, H. and Murillo-Llanes, J., 2012. Lack of effects of the TNF-alpha and IL-10 gene polymorphisms in Mexican patients with lepromatous leprosy. *Lepr. Rev.* 83, 34-9.

Walker, S. L. and Lockwood, D. N., 2008. Leprosy type 1 (reversal) reactions and their management. *Lepr. Rev.* 79, 372-86.

Wilson, A. G., di Giovine, F. S., Blakemore, A. I. and Duff, G. W., 1992. Single base polymorphism in the human tumour necrosis factor alpha (TNF alpha) gene detectable by NcoI restriction of PCR product. *Hum. Mol. Genet.* 1, 353.

Yilmaz, V., Yentur, S.P. and Saruhan-Direskeneli, G., 2005. IL-12 and IL-10 polymorphisms and their effects on cytokine production. *Cytokine* 30, 188-94.

In: Leprosy
Editor: Roger S. Kopp
ISBN: 978-1-63321-668-6

Chapter 2

In Vivo and *In Vitro* Evidence on the Relationship between Antiphospholipid Antibodies and Leprosy

***Ricardo Forastiero*[1,*] *and Marta Martinuzzo*[2]**
[1]Department of Physiology, Thrombosis and Hemostasis, Favaloro University,
[2]Central Laboratory, Italian Hospital of Buenos Aires, Buenos Aires, Argentina

Abstract

Leprosy is a chronic infection caused by *Mycobacterium Leprae*. The spectrum of clinical manifestations depends on different *Mycobacterium Leprae*-responsive T-cell subsets. Tuberculoid leprosy is associated with type 1 T helper cells, while T helper 2 cells are primarily associated with lepromatous leprosy (LL). LL is characterized by intense polyclonal activation of B lymphocytes resulting in multibacillary and disseminated disease, as well as development of a variety of autoantibodies. The antiphospholipid syndrome (APS) is an autoimmune disease that is

* Corresponding author: Ricardo Forastiero, Hematología, Universidad Favaloro, Solís 453, (C1078AAI) Buenos Aires, Argentina, Tel: +54 11 4378 1145, Fax: +54 11 4378 1311, e-mail: rforastiero@favaloro.edu.ar.

characterized serologically by the presence of antiphospholipid antibodies (aPL) and clinically by vascular thrombosis and/or recurrent pregnancy morbidity. The APS-associated aPL are mainly directed against β_2-glycoprotein I (β_2GPI) and prothrombin. On the other hand, aPL linked to infectious disorders are primarily directed against phospholipids and do not tend to be associated with the clinical manifestations of APS. This distinction, however, was found not to be absolute. Patients with LL present high prevalence of IgM aPL that bind β_2GPI, but they not develop thrombosis. Recent evidence suggests that APS autoantibodies to β_2GPI bind to critical epitopes in domain I, and leprosy-related aPL recognizing β_2GPI tend to be directed against domain V. The position of the epitope in the β_2GPI molecule seems to be critical for aPL pathogenicity in clinical manifestation of APS. It is accepted that aPL found in APS patients are themselves pathogenic. Patients with APS and those with LL show different *in vivo* cytokine profiles and circulating levels of tissue factor as well as differences in ongoing systemic coagulation and cellular activation. The most convincing support for the pathogenicity of aPL comes from animal models. In a murine model of thrombosis and endothelial cell activation we found that purified aPL reacting with β_2GPI from leprosy patients, in contrast to those from APS are not able to activate endothelium and to enhance thrombus formation *in vivo*. It could explain at least to some extent the different clinical behavior of patients with APS and leprosy-related aPL.

Introduction

Antiphospholipid antibodies (aPL) are a heterogeneous family of antibodies detected by different coagulation tests and immunologic assays. The diagnosis of lupus anticoagulant (LA) relies on a set of successive phospholipid-dependent clotting tests, and anticardiolipin (aCL) and anti-β_2 glycoprotein I antibodies (aβ_2GPI) are measured by different immunologic assays.Most LA are directed against either β_2GPI or prothrombin whereas antibodies detected in the aCL assay recognize β_2GPI complexed with cardiolipin or cardiolipin alone [1, 2].

Within the field of aPL there are two different and clear groups of patients. One includes subjects having an acute or chronic infection disorder and the other one include subjects with autoimmune disorders. aPL may bind phospholipids directly but most autoimmune aPL require β_2GPI and prothrombin for antibody binding to phospholipids. Positivity on the aCL assay not directed against β_2GPI is commonly found in the setting of several infectious disorders [2].

Since the 1980s, the term antiphospholipid syndrome (APS) is used to describe patients characterized clinically by the occurrence of objectively proven venous or arterial thrombosis in different vascular beds, and/or pregnancy morbidity in association to raised levels of aPL. Cerebrovascular infarction is the most common clinical feature within the arterial circulation, whereas lower limb deep venous thrombosis and pulmonary embolism are the main clinical manifestations within the venous circulation. The APS was firstly closely associated with systemic lupus erythematosus (SLE) but soon it was observed that this disorder is also found in patients in the absence of an underlying autoimmune disease. The 2006 updated criteria advises against using the expression secondary APS when APS is in the setting of autoimmune diseases. Rather than distinguishing between primary and secondary APS, documenting the coexistence of SLE (or other disease) with APS is suggested [1]. APS requires the combination of at least one clinical and one laboratory criterion. The recent consensus statement suggests avoiding classification of APS is less than 12 weeks or more than 5 years separate the positive aPL tests and the clinical manifestation. In addition, the evaluation of coexisting inherited and acquired thrombosis risk factors in APS patients is highly recommended. Consequently, patients fulfilling APS criteria must be stratified according to the presence or absence of contributing causes of thrombosis. The clinical criterion remains unchanged, but superficial venous thrombosis is now not included in the clinical criteria and transient cerebral ischemia and stroke are incorporated as presentations of vascular thrombosis. The consensus statement also state that livedo reticularis, cardiac valve disease, thrombocytopenia and nefropathy are features unquestionably common in patients with APS. However, they are not considered independent criteria for definite APS. From a clinical viewpoint, the new criteria are very useful in research and besides in real practice because they limit the inclusion of a diverse group of patients. In addition, the assessment of concurrent prothrombotic factors provides a risk-stratified approach that is in fact very important because some of them may be treatable [1].

The detection of persistently elevated levels of aPL is a requisite laboratory feature for the diagnosis of APS. The positivity for at least one aPL test: LA and/or IgG/IgM aCL (at titres higher than 40 units or the normal 99th percentile) and/or $a\beta_2$GPI (at titres higher than the normal 99th percentile) must be detected. They must be found on two or more occasions at least 12 weeks apart. In the 2006 updated APS criteria it is advised to classify APS patients in two different groups of categories. Patients with more than one positive aPL test must be placed in category I, while those with single aPL positivity must be placed in category II [3-7].

Syphilis was the first infection to be recognized as being linked to aPL. In addition, raised levels of aPL have been found in a large number of viral as well as bacterial infections, such as human immunodeficiency virus, hepatitis, tuberculosis, leprosy, cytomegalovirus, mycoplasma, Q fever, parvovirus, etc [8-10]. In most cases aCL disappear after resolution of the infectious disorder and the aPL titre is commonly low positive. IgM aCL are generally more prevalent than IgG aCL. LA activity is transient, weak and less frequently detected in comparison with aCL. In lepromatous leprosy (LL), however, LA is often detected and its activity is the strongest reported in infectious disorders [11]. Since the beginning, several authors have tried to find out differences between APS and infections-related aPL. Some differences in avidity binding to cardiolipin and other phospholipids, IgG subclasses, affinity, etc have been described. However, most findings remained controversial. aCL from infections and APS differ markedly in IgG subclass distribution. IgG_1 and IgG_3 were predominantly found in infections-related aCL, while IgG_2 and IgG_4 were the major subclasses of aPL associated with APS [12].

Leprosy is a chronic infectious disease caused by *Mycobacterium leprae*. Its broad spectrum of manifestations depends on the host immune response to the pathogen. Type 1 T helper (Th1) cells are associated with tuberculoid leprosy (TT), which is characterized by a protective response against the bacillus with effective control of the dissemination of the disease. In contrast, T helper 2 (Th2) cells are primarily associated with LL, which is characterized by intense polyclonal activation of B lymphocytes resulting in multibacillary and disseminated disease, as well as development of hypergammaglobulinaemia and autoantibodies. Between these extremes are immunologically unstable patients with intermediate signs and symptoms corresponding to the borderline tuberculoid (BT), mid-borderline (BB) and borderline lepromatous (BL) forms [13]. In 1982, the WHO established a simplified classification based on the bacterial index (BI). According to this classification, leprosy was divided into paucibacillary (PB) and multibacillary (MB). In 1988, the WHO recommended the use of a purely clinical classification because there are regions where microscopy examination of skin smear is unavailable, establishing as PB cases those patients with up to five skin lesions and/or only one nerve trunk involved, whereas MB cases are those with more than five skin lesions and/or more than one nerve trunk involved. However, when microscopy examination of skin smear is available, patients with positive results are considered MB, regardless of the number of lesions. Thus, indeterminate, TT and BT patients are included in the PB group. The MB group includes BB, BL, LL and some BT patients [14]. In this chapter, we will present the current knowledge on aPL linked to leprosy.

Prevalence of aPL in Leprosy

The presence of aPL in patients with leprosy has been recognized in many studies since 1986 [11, 12, 15-23]. The prevalence of LA, aCL, aβ_2GPI and anti-protrombin antibodies (aPT) varied among studies. Positivity rates were as high as 69 and 75% [11, 12]. aCL are the main antibodies evaluated showing a high prevalence in most studies (Table 1). Despite many case report publications, LA was only systematically investigated in two cases with a very different prevalence, 69 vs 10% in Argentinean [11] and Brazilian [16] studies, respectively. As described by de Larrañaga [11] all plasmas from patients which tested positive for LA had prolonged activated partial thromboplastin time, but 85.7% also had dilute Russell viper venom time positive, and in these plasmas aβ_2GPI and/or aPT were also detected. These findings suggested that LA in leprosy patients resembles those found in SLE or APS patients. The prevalence and aPL titre were found to be significantly more elevated in patients with LL than borderline forms and MB than in PB disease [12, 18, 19].

Considering the isotype, aCL were present as IgG and /or IgM, with different isotype profile among studies. de Larrañaga [11] and Ribeiro [20] found higher prevalence of IgM than IgG isotype in both aCL and aβ_2GPI of Argentinean and Brazilian leprosy patients, respectively. On the other hand, African patients studied by Arvieux [12] showed that both isotypes prevalence were similar. However, in other study the presence of both (IgG + IgM aCL) together was more frequent than any isolated isotype [18]. IgM aβ_2GPI were more common than IgG [11, 19-21], but IgG isotype was as prevalent as [12] or more prevalent than IgM aPT found in some series of patients [11].

The prevalence of IgG subclasses of aβ_2GPI and aPT expressed by patients with leprosy is peculiar and different to that observed in patients with APS [12]. Leprosy patients presented 89% of IgG_3 aβ_2GPI and 91% of IgG_3 aPT, but this subclass was only expressed by 14% and 13% of APS patients, respectively. On the other hand, IgG_2 is the main subclass expressed by APS patients, 100% for aβ_2GPI and aPT, compared to 33 and 45% by leprosy patients.

Table1. Prevalence of aPL in published series of patients with leprosy

Study	n	LA (%)	aCL IgG (%)	aCL IgM (%)	aCL IgG+IgM (%)	aβ_2GPI IgG (%)	aβ_2GPI IgM (%)	aβ_2GPI IgG+IgM (%)	aPT IgG (%)	aPT IgM (%)	aPT IgG+IgM (%)
Furukawa et al (1986)	45		20.0								
Thawani et al., (1994)	41 MB		19.5	4.8	60.9						
	43 PB		4.6	13.9	39.5						
Hojnik et al (1994)	61		96.7			18.0					
de Larrañaga et al., (2000)	51	68.6	2	43.1	15.7	2.0	51.0	3.9	27.4	7.8	9.8
Elbeialy et al., (2000)	35		37.0			2.9			5.7		
Arvieux et al., (2002)	176		10.2	17.6	10.8	13.6	13.6	11.9	11.4	14.8	15.3
Loizou et al., (2003)	112		7.1	4.5	0	8.0	28.6	48.2	8.0	2.7	1.8
Brochado et al., (2010)	67 MB					4.5	46.0				
	24 PB					0	17.0				
Ribeiro et al., (2011)	158		1.9	13.3	0.6	0.6	40.5	5.1			
Teixeira Junior et al., (2011)	100	10	3	11							

These differences may be due to the nature of antigen triggering antibody production, and it is in agreement with the association of increased IgG_1 and IgG_3 subclasses of antibodies anti-*M Leprae* and disease progression reported by Hussain [24].

Specificity of aPL in Leprosy Patients

Most sera from leprosy patients recognized human and bovine β_2GPI coated on plain polystyrene in the absence of cardiolipin [12], and inhibition of this binding was achieved when increased cardiolipin concentration was added to the first step coating, totally opposite to that observed in APS sera. The reason why aβ_2GPI occurring in leprosy and APS have different plate requirement in order to be detected in a direct ELISA may be related to their avidity. Additionally, some binding of leprosy but not APS antibodies was seen when cardiolipin alone in a β_2GPI-free assay was used, suggesting that true aCL can also be found in leprosy. These results were in agreement to those previously described [22], where different populations of aCL were present in patients with leprosy, some patients presenting β_2GPI-dependent and others β_2GPI-independent aCL. In addition, a small group of patients bound cardiolipin at the same extent either in presence or absence of β_2GPI.

It has been demonstrated that aCL and aβ_2GPI activities present in sera from leprosy and from APS patients showed the same degree of inhibition when they were incubated with liposomes containing cardiolipin and β_2GPI [11]. However, when fluid-phase inhibition experiments with *Mycobacterium Leprae* lysates where performed the aCL binding was inhibited, but aβ_2GPI reactivity was unchanged, indicating that true aβ_2GPI were present in leprosy sera.

Moreover, it was demonstrated that aβ_2GPI found in leprosy can bind β_2GPI coated in plain polystyrene plates (without irradiation, condition needed for APS aβ_2GPI binding). This binding cannot be inhibited by preincubation with a monoclonal antibody that binds domain I of β_2GPI as occurred with APS sera, and they have greater avidity than APS aβ_2GPI as demonstrated by β_2GPI fluid-phase inhibition studies. Additionally, antibodies present in leprosy can bind deleted mutants of domain I (DM II-V) and V (DM I-IV) in the same extent as the whole molecule of β_2GPI. On the other hand, most APS antibodies recognized DM I-IV but failed to bind DM II-V, indicating that epitope recognized by APS and leprosy aβ_2GPI are different [12].

A very nice work performed by Panunto-Castelo [25] demonstrated that Rubino reaction (RR), that was considered a test very specific for diagnosis of leprosy patients with defective *Mycobacterium Leprae*-specific cell immunity, was mediated by an aβ_2GPI that bound to β_2GPI coupled to membrane phospholipids expressed on the surface of formalynized sheep red-blood cells (FSRBC). The purified IgM could bind the surface of FSRBC only in the presence of β_2GPI as a cofactor by means of flow cytometry and inmunoblotting studies. The component present in the FSRBC needed for leprosy patients IgM binding was lost when cells were treated with methanol/chloroform, and thus confirming that was a lipid by thin layer chromatography. Thus the Rubino test for leprosy is a β_2GPI-dependent anti-phospholipid reaction. Even more, the RR was positive in 45% of sera from patients with SLE and high titre of aCL, demonstrating that this test was not specific for leprosy and that autoimmune aPL produce false positive results.

A very interesting observation about aβ_2GPI production in leprosy patients was done by a Brazilian group [19[. They analysed the presence of 4 single-nucleotide polymorphisms (SNPs) of the β_2GPI gene: Ser88Asn, Leu247Val, Cys306Gly and Trp316Ser in 113 leprosy patients. They found that only Leu247Val polymorphism (Val/Val homozygocity) was more prevalent in leprosy patients than in controls, and that this homozygocity was associated to the presence of aβ_2GPI IgM in this series. Moreover, when seven patients with thrombotic manifestations were analyzed, there were 3 homozygous and 4 heterozygous, suggesting a possible association of the β_2GPI genotype with the infrequent APS manifestations in these patients,

Do aPL Positive Leprosy Patients Share Páthogenic Mechanisms with APS Patients?

Many groups found that patients with leprosy very frequently developed aCL, aβ_2GPI and/or LA but do not present clinical features of APS [11, 12, 17, 20, 21] or described very few patients with thrombosis [19, 26, 27].These findings prompted us to evaluate some pathogenic mechanisms in this group of patients [28]. We demonstrated in previous studies that a state of platelet activation *in vivo* is present in patients with aPL reflected by the increased urinary levels of 11-dehydro thromboxane B_2 of platelet origin, and this effect was related to the presence of aβ_2GPI [29]. In the same way it has been proved that aβ_2GPI activate platelets *in vitro* and different mechanisms mediating these effects have been described [30-33]. We demonstrated that soluble P selectin (sPSel) levels were elevated in aPL (+) leprosy patients as well as in patients with APS, compared to controls and aPL (-) leprosy [28], demonstrating that platelet activation *ex vivo* was a common mechanism related to the presence of aPL, even in leprosy patients.

The expression of adhesion molecules on endothelial cells (EC) directs the cellular traffic to sites of inflammation. VCAM-1 (vascular cell adhesion molecule 1) is present on EC activated by cytokines, but it could also be expressed by lymphocytes and monocytes. Binding of autoimmune aPL and aβ_2GPI to EC surface has been shown to lead to cell activation increasing the expression of adhesion molecules including VCAM-1, in *in vitro* experiments and in animal models [34, 35]. We and other authors have previously showed that soluble markers of EC activation were elevated in patients with aPL and APS [36, 37]. We also observed that aPL (+) leprosy patients (all LL) had increased levels of sVCAM-1 compared to either normal controls or aPL (-) leprosy patients, and in the same extent as seen in APS patients. However some aPL(-) leprosy patients presented also elevated levels of sVCAM-1 probably due to the strong cellular immune mediated response involved in this disease [28]. There is a report about the significance of soluble levels of intercellular adhesion molecule-1 (ICAM-1) and E selectin as markers of disease activity in 74 patients with leprosy. Both soluble adhesion molecules were elevated in lepromatous compared to tuberculoid type and healthy controls, but aPL were not investigated in this group of patients [38]. Interestingly they found that levels of soluble ICAM-1 and E selectin dropped after anti mycobacterial treatment correlating with mycobacteria loaded reduction in skin biopsies. In our study we could not correlate levels of soluble VCAM-1 and E selectin with treatment because all the evaluated patients were on treatment or vigilance.

A procoagulant state has been suggested by the *in vivo* up-regulation of tissue factor pathway in patients with APS and history of thrombosis [39]. We found increased levels of markers of blood coagulation activation such as prothrombin F1+2 fragment (F1+2) and thrombin-antithrombin complexes (TAT) in patients with aPL, even in patients who were under oral anticoagulant treatment, although to a lesser extent [36]. In contrast, leprosy patients presented normal levels of both markers regardless of the presence of aPL [28], although D dimer (DD) levels were scattered and they were slightly elevated in some leprosy patients either with or without aPL, and clearly lower than patients with APS.

It is also well recognized that aPL interfere with the activity of activated protein C (PC) and that the effect is mainly due to aβ_2GPI [40]. We found a lower prevalence of interference with the PC pathway (measured by using the ProC global test) in aPL(+) leprosy patients as compared to a control group of autoimmune aPL patients [28]. This finding could only partially explain the normal results of F1+2 and TAT observed in our cohort of leprosy patients with aPL. We cannot exclude a haemostatic abnormality that could contribute to the inhibition of systemic coagulation activation. Different epitopes recognized by aβ_2GPI present in leprosy and APS patients could be important in this way.

As a consequence of EC and monocyte activation, tissue factor (TF) expression on the surface of these cells is highly increased. The combination of upregulation of TF and decreased TF pathway inhibitor (TFPI) activity has been largely demonstrated in patients with APS, thus contributing to the hypercoagulable state in this disorder [41-44]. It could be, at least in part, responsible for the procoagulant state, as evidenced by increased levels of F1+2 and TAT, observed in APS patients but not in patients with leprosy related aPL. Raised plasma levels of soluble TF (sTF) have been shown in APS patients, although the cell origin of sTF and its importance as an accurate marker of systemic TF pathway remain unclear [41-43]. Inflammatory mediators like tumour necrosis factor (TNF-α) and interleukin 6 (IL-6) are able to perturb the haemostatic balance, thus triggering coagulation [45, 46]. In a previous study, we found that patients with autoimmune aPL and a diagnosis of primary APS show a predominance of Th2-type response, as evidenced by a significant increase in serum levels of IL-6 and a decrease of interferon γ (IFN- γ) and IL-2 [47].

In a recent study, circulating levels of tissue factor and proinflammatory cytokines were evaluated in patents with APS, asymptomatic aPL patients and leprosy [48]. The study recruited 42 patients with APS without underlying SLE, 42 subjects with persistent autoimmune aPL (non-APS group) and 48 with leprosy (40 LL and 8 BL). A trend to higher sTF levels was found in patients with autoimmune aPL. Furthermore, the prevalence of high sTF plasma levels was significantly greater not only in patients with primary APS but also in those from the non-APS group. These findings could partly explain previous data showing that an ongoing prothrombotic state, as evidenced by increased levels of markers of blood coagulation activation, is observed in both aPL patients with or without clinical features of definite APS. sTF plasma concentration significantly correlated with titres of IgG aCL or IgG aβ_2GPI in patients with previous venous thrombosis. Despite exhibiting high prevalence of conventional aPL as well as aβ_2GPI and aPT, leprosy patients (with or without aPL) included in that study did not show high levels of sTF. This observation could be compatible with a previous work, in which leprosy patients presented normal levels of markers of blood coagulation activation regardless of the presence of aPL. Some data could account for the different *in vivo* behaviour of TF in APS and leprosy. Leprosy related aPL differ from APS related ones with respect to the predominant immunoglobulin isotype, avidity and epitope specificity of aβ_2GPI. The absence of antibodies to TFPI in leprosy could also contribute to explain the different prothrombotic state seen in APS and leprosy [49].

It is now accepted that the cytokine network triggers cascades of reactions and multiple responses representing an important link between inflammation and coagulation [45, 46, 50]. Most inflammatory mediators upregulate certain prothrombotic pathways as well as downregulate some anticoagulant ones. The balance between Th1 and Th2 cells and the rise of Th2 related cytokines (IL-6 and IL-4) was associated with an important role in the development of APS in mice [51]. Decreased IFN-γ/IL-6 ratios attributable to high IL-6 and a trend to lower IFN-γ production were found in definite APS patients. In opposition, enhanced ratios reflecting elevated IFN-γ and normal IL-6 were observed in leprosy patients [48]. IL-6 is mostly produced by fibroblasts, monocytes and T- and B-lymphocytes. Elevated levels of IL-6 have been associated with recurrent venous thrombosis and activation of coagulation and platelets. The bioactivity of IL-6 is enhanced in the presence of its agonist, sIL-6R (soluble IL-6 receptor), which renders cells only expressing the membrane bound glycoprotein 130 responsive towards the cytokine IL-6. There was a positive correlation between sIL-6R and IL-6 only in patients with autoimmune aPL suggesting that the IL-6-mediated inflammatory effects could be more effective in APS patients than in leprosy. Leprosy patients with or without aPL had the highest values of TNF-α, but IL-6 and TNF-α correlated to a smaller degree than in APS [48]. This could in part explain that leprosy patients with aPL show platelet and EC activation *in vivo* to the same extent than APS patients. As a whole, raised serum levels of proinflammatory cytokines such as IL-6 and TNF-α are found in patients with definite primary APS. Leprosy patients with aPL, however, have increased TNF-α but normal IL-6 levels. The different cytokine profiles as well as differences in circulating levels of TF might contribute to the high thrombotic risk found in patients with autoimmune aPL but not in leprosy related aPL patients. A summary of the different pathogenic effects observed in aPL patients with either leprosy or APS is shown in Table 2.

Table 2. Main contrasting effects or characteristics between aPL from APS or leprosy

	Leprosy	APS
Binding to		
Domain I of β_2GPI	no	yes
Domain V of β_2GPI	yes	no
Plasma levels of soluble		
prothrombin fragment 1 + 2	Normal	High
thrombin–antithrombin complexes	Normal	High
D dimer	Normal	High
tissue factor	Normal	High
P selectin	High	High
VCAM-1	High	High
TNF-α	High	High
IL-6	Normal	High
IL-6 receptor	Normal	Normal
IFN-γ	High	Low
Effects in *in vivo* animal models		
thrombogenic	no	yes
pro-inflammatory	no	yes

In Vivo Studies Linking aPL with Leprosy

As mentioned before, patients with leprosy present high frequency and elevated titres of IgM aβ_2GPI, but they do not develop thrombosis. There is convincing evidence that aPL/aβ_2GPI from APS are pathogenic *in vivo* and *in vitro* [52, 53]. The most conclusive support for the pathogenicity of aPL comes from different murine models. The murine pinch-induced thrombosis model and the leukocyte adhesion to endothelium in the microcirculation model of the cremaster muscle have been extensively used to evaluate the thrombogenic and pro-inflammatory effects of aPL purified from APS patients. The passive administration of polyclonal and monoclonal antibdies from APS patients to mice has been an important model in establishing that IgG, IgM and also IgA aPL do display biological properties *in vivo* that can lead to thrombotic events, thus supporting its pathogenicity in humans [54, 55].

In a recent paper, we used the same murine model of thrombosis and endothelial cell activation to compare the thrombogenic and pro-inflammatory effects of IgM purified from leprosy with those from APS patients [56]. Sera from patients with APS or with lepromatous leprosy were used as the source of IgM antibodies. All patients with APS had strong LA activity, and high titres of IgM aCL and aβ_2GPI. All APS patients had a history of venous thrombosis and/or cerebrovascular accidents. Among the leprosy patients, all but one had strong LA activity, and high titres of IgM aCL and aβ_2GPI. None of the leprosy patients had evidence of APS-related clinical features. CD1 mice were treated at 0 hours and 48 hours later with IgM aPL with high titre of aβ_2GPI isolated from patients with leprosy or APS or with IgM from healthy controls or leprosy aPL negative control. Seventy-two hours after the first injection, the adhesion of leukocytes (#WBC) to EC in cremaster muscle (as an indication of EC activation *in vivo*), as well as the size of an induced thrombus in the femoral vein of the mice were examined.

There were differences on the dynamics of thrombus formation between mice immunized with IgM APS preparations and IgM normal controls. The median thrombus size was significantly larger in the group immunized with IgM APS compared with IgM controls. Moreover, median thrombus area was significantly larger in mice injected with IgM APS compared with IgM isolated from aPL positive or negative leprosy. Median thrombus sizes in IgM leprosy, IgM leprosy control and IgM healthy controls were not significantly different. Regarding the *in vivo* microcirculation murine model, mice injected with IgM APS had significantly more leukocyte adhering to endothelium in cremaster muscle than those injected with IgM preparations from the other 3 groups. Mice immunized with IgM leprosy (aPL positive or negative) had a slightly lower number of endothelium-adhering WBC than IgM healthy controls.

These findings about IgM preparations from APS patients are in agreement with the previous findings that not only IgG but also IgM aPL are able to increase the thrombus formation in an *in vivo* animal model. Our data clearly show that aPL/aβ_2GPI from leprosy patients do not show thrombogenic and pro-inflammatory effects *in vivo* when compared with aPL derived from APS [56].

Recent studies have shown that thrombogenic aβ_2GPI are mainly directed against domain I of β_2GPI, whereas aβ_2GPI directed to other domains of the molecule do not seem to be pathogenic. In a recent publication, recombinant domain I of β_2GPI inhibited the aPL-induced enhancement of *in vivo* thrombosis in a dose-dependent manner [57]. It has been reported that antibodies targeting β_2GPI from leprosy mainly bind to domain V of β_2GPI. Therefore, the *in vivo* results are in accordance with previous data indicating that although patients with leprosy present a very high prevalence of aPL, they do not show a procoagulant state. The data support the findings that not all aβ_2GPI are pathogenic and it is possible that in lepromatous leprosy patients the aβ_2GPI found in their serum recognize other domains of the molecule. Leprosy patients could have the 'innocent' profile of aβ_2GPI as reported in a recent publication [58].

Conclusion

aPL are present in a variety of diseases including autoimmune and infectious disorders. According to findings in the last years, not all aPL are pathogenic. Most aPL associated with thrombosis recognise certain phospholipid-binding proteins such as β_2GPI and prothrombin. On the other hand, the majority of infection-linked aPL are mainly directed against phospholipids. However, leprosy-related aPL resemble APS antibodies because most aPL found in leprosy do recognise β_2GPI. Nevertheless, despite similar aPL laboratory profile leprosy and APS patients greatly differ in clinical features. Thrombosis is one of the main APS clinical criteria but it is rarely found in the setting of leprosy patients with aPL. Data coming from diverse *in vitro* and *in vivo* studies have tried to clarify this fact. Likely some differences in antibody properties (avidity, isotype, and epitope specificity) may explain the contrasting clinical features found in patients with leprosy or APS.

References

[1] Miyakis, S, Lockshin MD, Atsumi T, Branch DW, Brey RL, Cervera R, Derksen RH, de Groot PG, Koike T, Meroni PL, Reber G, Shoenfeld Y, Tincani A, Vlachoyiannopoulos PG, Krilis SA. International consensus statement on an update of the classification criteria for definite antiphospholipid syndrome (APS). *J. Thromb. Haemost.* 2006; 4: 295-306.

[2] Forastiero R, Martinuzzo M. Antigen specificity and clinical relevance of antiphospholipid syndrome-related autoantibodies. *Curr. Rheumatol. Rev.* 2005; 1: 177-187.

[3] Forastiero R. Trends in the antiphospholipid syndrome criteria. *J. Hematol. Thromb. Dis.* 2013; 1: 1-2.

[4] Pengo V, Banzato A, Denas G, Jose SP, Bison E, Hoxha A, Ruffatti A. Correct laboratory approach to APS diagnosis and monitoring. *Autoimmun. Rev.* 2013; 12: 832-834.

[5] Forastiero R, Papalardo E, Watkins M, Nguyen H, Quirbach C, Jaskal K, Kast M, Teodorescu M, Lakos G, Binder W, Shums Z, Nelson V, Norman G, Puig J, Cox A, Vandam W, Hardy J, Pierangeli S. Evaluation *Clin. Chim. Acta* 2014; 428: 99-105.

[6] de Laat B, Derksen RH, Urbanus RT, de Groot PG. IgG antibodies that recognize epitope Gly40-Arg43 in domain I of beta 2-glycoprotein I cause LAC, and their presence correlates strongly with thrombosis. *Blood* 2005; 105: 1540-1545.

[7] de Laat B, de Groot PG. Autoantibodies directed domain I of beta2-glycoprotein I. *Curr. Rheumatol. Rep.* 2011; 13: 70-76.

[8] Gharavi AE, Pierangeli SS, Harris EN. Origin of antiphospholipid antibodies. Rheum. *Dis. Clin. North Am.* 2001; 27: 551-563.

[9] Gharavi AE, Pierangeli SS, Harris EN. Viral origin of antiphospholipid antibodies: endothelial cell activation and thrombus enhancement by CMV peptide-induced APL antibodies. *Immunobiology* 2003; 207: 37-42.

[10] Santiago M, Martinelli R, Ko A, Reis EA, Fontes RD, Nascimento EG, Pierangeli S, Espinola R, Gharavi A. Anti-beta2 glycoprotein I and anticardiolipin antibodies in leptospirosis, syphilis and Kala-azar. *Clin. Exp. Rheumatol.* 2001; 19: 425-430.

[11] de Larrañaga G, Forastiero RR, Martinuzzo ME, Carreras LO, Tsariktsian G, Sturno MM, Alonso BS. High prevalence of antiphospholipid antibodies in leprosy: evaluation of antigen reactivity. *Lupus* 2000; 9: 594-600.

[12] Arvieux J, Renaudineau Y, Mane I, Perraut R, Krilis SA, Youinou P. Distinguishing features of anti-β_2 glycoprotein I antibodies between patients with leprosy and the antiphospholipid syndrome. *Thromb Haemost.* 2002; 87: 599-605.

[13] Ridley D, Jopling M. Classification of leprosy according to immunity. A five-group system. Int J Lep Other Mycobact Dis. 1966; 34: 255-273.

[14] Lastória JC, Abreu MA. Leprosy: review of the epidemiological, clinical, and etiopathogenic aspects - Part 1. *An. Bras. Dermatol.* 2014; 89: 205-218.

[15] Furukawa F, Kashihara M, Imamura S, Ohshio G, Hamashima Y. Evaluation *Acta Dermatol. Res.* 1986; 278: 317-319.
[16] Teixeira Junior GJ, Silva CE, Magalhães V. Application of the diagnostic criteria for systemic lupus erythematosus to patients with multibacillary leprosy. *Rev. Soc. Bras. Med. Trop.* 2011; 44: 85-90.
[17] Elbeialy A, Strassburger-Lorna K, Atsumi T, Bertolaccini ML, Amengual O, Hanafi M, Khamashta MA, Hughes GR. Antiphospholipid antibodies in leprotic patients: a correlation *Clin. Exp. Rheumatol.* 2000; 18: 492-494.
[18] Thawani G, Bhatia VN, Mukherjee A. Anticardiolipin antibodies in leprosy *Indian J. Lepr.* 1994; 66: 307-314.
[19] Brochado MJ, Figueiredo JF, Mendes-Junior CT, Louzada-Junior P, Kim O, Roselino AM. Correlation between beta-2-glycoprotein I gene polymorphism and anti-beta-2 glycoprotein I antibodies in patients with multibacillary leprosy. *Arch. Dermatol. Res.* 2010; 302: 583–591.
[20] Ribeiro SLE, Pereira HLA, Silva NP, Souza AWS, Sato EI. Anti-β_2-glycoprotein I antibodies are highly prevalent in a large number of Brazilian leprosy patients. *Acta Reumatol. Port* 2011, 36: 30-37.
[21] Loizou S, Singh S, Wypkema E, Asherson RA. Anticardiolipin, anti-β_2-glycoprotein I and antiprothrombin antibodies in black South African patients with infectious disease. *Ann. Rheum. Dis.* 2003; 62: 1106-1111.
[22] Hojnik M, Gilburd B, Ziporen L, Blank M, Tomer Y, Scheinberg MA, Tincani A, Rozman B, Shoenfeld Y. Anticardiolipin antibodies in infections are heterogeneous in their dependency on beta 2-glycoprotein I: analysis of anticardiolipin *Lupus* 1994; 3: 515-521.
[23] Guedes Barbosa LS, Gilbrut B, Shoenfeld Y, Scheinberg MA. Autoantibodies in leprosy sera. *Clin. Rheumatol.* 1996; 15: 26-28.
[24] Hussain R, Kifayet A, Chiang TJ. Immunoglobulin G1 (lgG1) and IgG3 antibodies are markers of progressive disease in leprosy. *Infect. Immun.* 1995; 63: 410-415.
[25] Panunto-Castelo A, Almeida IC, Rosa JC, Greene LJ, Roque-Barreira MC. The Rubino test for leprosy is a β_2-glycoprotein 1-dependent antiphospholipid reaction. *Immunol.* 2000; 101: 147-153.
[26] Bakos L, Correa CC, Bergmann L, Bonamigo RR, Muller LF. Antiphospholipid antibodies thrombotic syndrome misdiagnosed as Lucio's phenomenon. *Int. J. Lepr. Other Mycobact. Dis.* 1996; 64: 320-323.
[27] Akerkar SM, Bichile LS. Leprosy & gangrene: a rare association; role of anti phospholipid antibodies. *BMC Infect. Dis.* 2005; 5: 74.

[28] Martinuzzo ME, de Larrañaga GF, Forastiero RR, Pelegri Y, Fariña MH, Alonso BS, Kordich LC, Carreras LO. Markers of platelet, endothelial cell and blood coagulation activation markers in leprosy patients with antiphospholipid antibodies. *Clin. Exp. Rheumatol.* 2002; 20: 477-483.

[29] Forastiero RR, Martinuzzo ME, Carreras LO, Maclouf J. Anti- b2 glycoprotein I antibodies and platelet activation in patients with antiphospholipid antibodies: association with increased excretion of platelet-derived thromboxane urinary metabolites. *Thromb Haemost.* 1998; 79: 42-45.

[30] Martinuzzo ME, Maclouf J, Carreras LO, Lévy Toledano S. Antiphospholipid antibodies enhance thrombin-induced platelet activation and thromboxane formation. *Thromb Haemost.* 1993; 70: 667-671.

[31] Shi T, Giannakopoulos B, Yan X, Yu P, Berndt MC, Andrews RK, Rivera J, Iverson GM, Cockerill KA, Linnik MD, Krilis SA. Anti-beta2-glycoprotein I antibodies in complex with beta2-glycoprotein I can activate platelets in a dysregulated manner via glycoprotein Ib-IX-V. *Arthritis Rheum.* 2006; 54: 2558-2567.

[32] van Lummel M, Pennings MT, Derksen RH, Urbanus RT, Lutters BC, Kaldenhoven N, de Groot PG. The binding site in {beta)2-glycoprotein I for ApoER2' on platelets is located in domain V. *J. Biol. Chem.* 2005; 280: 36729-36736.

[33] Vega-Ostertag M, Harris EN, Pierangeli SS. Intracellular events in platelet activation induced by antiphospholipid antibodies in the presence of low doses of thrombin._*Arthritis Rheum.* 2004; 50: 2911-2919.

[34] Simantov R, LaSala JM, Lo SK, Gharavi AE, Sammaritano LR, Salmon JE, Silverstein RL. Activation of cultured vascular endothelial cells by antiphospholipid antibodies. *J. Clin. Invest.* 1995; 96: 2211-2219.

[35] Pierangeli S, Colden-Stanfield M, Liu X, Barker J, Anderson G, Harris E. Antiphospholipid antibodies from antiphospholipid syndrome patients activate endothelial cells *in vitro* and *in vivo*. *Circulation* 1999; 99: 1997-2002.

[36] Martinuzzo ME, Forastiero RR, Kordich L, Carreras LO. Increased lipid peroxidation correlates with platelet activation but not with markers of endothelial cell and blood coagulation activation in patients with antiphospholipid antibodies. *Br. J. Haematol.* 2001, 114: 845-51.

[37] Kaplanski G, Cacoub P, Farnarier C, Marin V, Grégoire R, Gatel A, Durand JM, Harlé JR, Bongrand P, Piette JC. Increased soluble vascular

cell adhesion molecule 1 concentrations in patients with primary or systemic lupus erythematosus -related antiphospholipid syndrome. *Arthritis Rheum.* 2000; 43: 55-64.

[38] Rieckmann P, Scholze G, Weichselbraun I, Ganapati R, Prange HW. Soluble adhesion molecules in sera of patients with leprosy: levels of soluble intercellular adhesion molecule-1 (sICAM-1) rapidly decrease during multi-drug therapy. *Clin. Exp. Immunol.* 1996; 105: 65-68.

[39] López-Pedrera C, Buendía P, Aguirre MA, Velasco F, Cuadrado MJ. Antiphospholipid syndrome and tissue factor: a thrombotic couple. *Lupus* 2006; 15: 161-166.

[40] De Groot PG, Derksen RHWM. The influence of antiphospholipid antibodies on the protein C pathway. *In* KHAMASHTA MA(Ed): *Hughes Syndrome. Antiphospholipid Syndrome.* London, Springer Press 2000: 307-315.

[41] Amengual O, Atsumi T, Khamashta MA, Hughes GRV. The role of the tissue factor pathway in the hypercoagulable state in patients with the antiphospholipid syndrome. *Thromb Haemost.* 1998; 79: 276–281.

[42] Dobado-Berrios P, Lopez-Pedrera C, Velasco F, Cuadrado MJ. The role of tissue factor in the antiphospholipid syndrome. *Arthritis Rheum.* 2001; 44: 2467–2476.

[43] Williams FMK, Parmar K, Hughes GRV, Hunt BJ. Systemic endothelial cell markers in primary antiphospholipid syndrome. *Thromb Haemost.* 2000; 84: 742–746.

[44] Forastiero RR, Martinuzzo ME, Broze GJ. High titres of autoantibodies to tissue factor pathway inhibitor are associated with the antiphospholipid syndrome. *J. Thromb Haemost.* 2003; 1: 718–724.

[45] Grignani G, Maiolo A. Cytokines and hemostasis. *Haematologica* 2000; 85: 967–972.

[46] Esmon CT. Does inflammation contribute to thrombotic events? *Haemostasis* 2000; 30: 34–40.

[47] Forastiero R, Martinuzzo M, Carreras LO. Imbalance towards Th2-type response in patients with definite primary antiphospholipid syndrome. *Thromb Haemost.* 2001; 86: 934–935.

[48] Forastiero RR, Martinuzzo ME, de Larrañaga G. Circulating levels of tissue factor and proinflammatory cytokines in patients with primary antiphospholipid syndrome or leprosy-related antiphospholipid antibodies. *Lupus* 2005; 14: 129-136.

[49] Forastiero R, Martinuzzo M, de Larrañaga G, Broze G. Antibodies to tissue factor pathway inhibitor are uncommonly detected in patients with

infection-related antiphospholipid antibodies. *J. Thromb Haemost.* 2003; 1: 2250-2251.

[50] Levi M, van der Poll T, Schultz M. New insights into pathways that determine the link between infection and thrombosis. *J. Med.* 2012; 70: 114-120.

[51] Krause I, Blank M, Levi Y, Koike T, Barak V, Shoenfeld Y. Anti-idiotype immunomodulation of experimental anti-phospholipid syndrome via effect on Th1/Th2 expression. *Clin. Exp. Immunol.* 1999; 117: 190–197.

[52] Aguilar-Valenzuela R, Martínez-Martínez LA, Pierangeli SS.A comprehensive review of thrombogenic mechanisms in APS. The Open Autoimmun J2010; 2: 58-66.

[53] Giannakopoulos B, Passam F, Rahgozar S, Krilis SA. Current concepts on the pathogenesis of the antiphospholipid syndrome. *Blood* 2007; 109: 422-430.

[54] Pierangeli S, Liu X, Barker J, Anderson G, Harris E. Induction of thrombosis in a mouse model by IgG, IgM and IgA immunoglobulins from patients with the antiphospholipid syndrome. *Thromb Haemost.* 1995; 74: 1361-1367.

[55] Pierangeli S, Colden-Stanfield M, Liu X, Barker J, Anderson G, Harris E. Antiphospholipid antibodies from antiphospholipid syndrome patients activate endothelial cells *in vitro* and *in vivo*. *Circulation* 1999; 99: 1997-2002.

[56] Forastiero R, Martinuzzo M, de Larrañaga G, Vega-Ostertag M, Pierangeli S. Anti-β_2-glycoprotein I antibodies from leprosy patients do not show thrombogenic effects in an *in vivo* animal model. *J. Thromb Haemost.* 2011, 9: 859-861.

[57] Ioannou Y, Romay-Penabad Z, Periclerous C, Giles I, Papalardo E, Vargas G, Shilagard T, Latcham DS, Isenberg DA, Rahman A, Pierangeli S. *In vivo* inhibition of antibody-induced pathogenicity utilizing the antigenic target peptide domain I of β_2-glycoprotein I: proof of concept. *J. Thromb Haemost.* 2009; 7: 833-842.

[58] Andreoli L, Nalli C, Motta M, Norman GL, Shums Z, Encabo S, Binder WL, Nuzzo M, Frassi M, Lojacono A, Avcin T, Meroni PL, Tincani A. Anti-beta2-glycoprotein I IgG antibodies from 1-year-old healthy children born to mothers with systemic autoimmune diseases preferentially target domain 4/5: might it be the reason for their 'innocent' profile? *Ann. Rheum. Dis.* 2011; 70: 380-383.

In: Leprosy
Editor: Roger S. Kopp

ISBN: 978-1-63321-668-6

Chapter 3

Leprosy and Pregnancy: A Epidemiological and Social Study in the Pará State, North of Brazil

Vera Regina da Cunha Menezes Palácios[1,*], Cléa Nazaré Carneiro Bichara[2], Régis Bruni Andriolo[3], Mauro José Pantoja Fonteles[4], Brenda Nazaré Gomes Andriolo[5], Nélson Veiga Gonçalves[6] and Marinete Marins Póvoa[7]

[1]Doctor in Biology of Infectious and Parasitic Agents at the Federal University of Pará (UFPA), Physician in Dermatologist, Coordinator in the Program of Medical Internship in Family Medicine of the State University of Pará (UEPA), Chief of the Communitarian Health Department (UEPA), Brazil

[2]Doctor in Biology of Infectious and Parasitic Agents at the Federal University of Pará (UFPA), Physician in infectious diseases, Professor of graduation and post graduation in medicine (M.D. and Ph.D.) at UEPA, Brazil

* Vera Regina da Cunha Menezes Palácios, Email: verareginapalacios@gmail.com, Fones: 55 (91) 99 83 30 13, 55 (91) 84 21 53 51, 55 (91) 3230 25 44.

[3]Doctor in Medicine based in Evidence at the Federal University of São Paulo (UNIFESP), Biologist, Professor of graduation and post graduation in medicine (M.D. and Ph.D.) at UEPA, Brazil

[4]Doctor in surgery at State University of Campinas (UNICAMP-São Paulo), Surgeon physician, Professor of graduation and post graduation in medicine (M.D. and Ph.D.) at UEPA, Brazil

[5]Doctor in Medicine based in Evidence at the Federal University of São Paulo (UNIFESP), Physiotherapist, Professor of graduation in medicine at UEPA, Brazil

[6]Doctor in Information Science at Nacional University of Brasilia (UNB), Epidemiologist, Professor of graduation and post graduation in medicine (M.D. and Ph.D.) at UEPA, Brazil, Professor at Rural Federal University of the Amazon (UFRA), Brazil

[7]Doctor in Medical Parasitology, University of London, Researcher at Evandro Chagas Institute (IEC), Pharmaceutics and biochemistry a t Universidade Federal Fluminense do Rio de Janeiro, Brazil

Abstract

Leprosy is still a big social and public health problem in many countries. Brazil has been for years in the second worldwide position in incidence and prevalence, after India in this ranking. Among the nearly five thousand Brazilian counties, 252 are priorities for actions to control and prevent of this disease. The highest prevalence occurs in the north region due to intense migratory flows and poverty. In the Amazon 35% of Brazilian cases are notified, currently the state of Pará is one of the major representative of the region. Leprosy associated with pregnancy is uncommon, with few and old publications about the theme. The Lucio's phenomenon was observed as the most frequent association complication in the last trimester of pregnancy, when there is an increase in depression of cellular immunity. The aim of this study was to analyze the epidemiological situation of this association by counties and Integration Regions (IR) in Pará State, from 2007 to 2009. Epidemiological and socio-demographic data obtained from the database of the National System of Notifiable Diseases, of the Ministry of Health, Pará State Health Department and Brazilian Institute of Geography and Statistics were analyzed. An epidemiologic indicator was developed to calculate the Detection Coefficient of the Association between Leprosy and Pregnancy (DCLP) also statistical and spatial analysis were performed through the percentile and Kernel methods in order to create the parameters of endemicity needed to evaluate the magnitude of the association and its distribution in each county of the state of Pará, taking into consideration socioeconomic characteristics. As a result it was observed that in 2007, 2008 and 2009 the DCLP was equal to 0,31 with 7 hyperendemic counties, 0,30 with 5 counties and 0,19 with 2 hyperendemic counties, respectively. Eldorado dos Carajás and Conceição do Araguaia, both in the southeast of the state had the highest coefficient of detection in the period (5,7 per 10.000 inhabitants) and a "very high" standard within the three years of study, respectively. Despite CDHGs have shown in most counties endemic pattern as "low" and decreasing year by year, in the studied period the unsatisfactory results of the analysis of social and epidemiological variables showed that the surveillance system has been ineffective in achieving the goal of the Organization World Health Organization (WHO), which is to reduce the prevalence of leprosy to less than one case per 10,000 inhabitants. The interpretation of the parameters of DCLP enabled the generation of qualiquantitative analysis, allowing to draw the socio-epidemiological panorama of the association, making the coefficient developed a new and useful analysis tool, because the informational contents produced may be used in planning processes and adoption of more efficient measures of surveillance and control of the disease, mitigating its social consequences.

Keywords: Leprosy, pregnancy, epidemiology

Introduction

Leprosy is still a major public health problem in the world. In 2012, for instance; 105 countries have still reported it to the World Health Organization (WHO). India and Brazil were the most prevalent within these countries. Although *detection rates* have fallen down every year, which translates a downward trend, this fall has been away from what one can expect [1].

Leprosy seems to have emerged in Asia, ranging from India to China and is believed to have been brought to the Mediterranean by the conquests of Alexander the Great (king of Macedonia) and from there to Europe and Americas [2].

'World Day to fight against Leprosy' was instituted in 1954, on the last Sunday of January, aiming at drawing world attention to that problem. This Public Health Aid challenge still continues in many countries throughout the 21st century. In Europe, leprosy virtually disappeared, except in Portugal,

Spain and Italy. Brazil has still been included in the position of endemic country, because it shows the highest rate in the Americas [2].

Concept and Etiology

Leprosy is a chronic, infectious and contagious, chronic, granulomatous, and millennial disease caused by *Mycobacterium leprae (M. leprae)*: An alcohol-acid resistant bacillus, compulsory intracellular parasite and its interaction with humans results in different clinical manifestations with varied signs and symptoms from several phisiopathological causes. It is now a curable disease through multidrug multichemotherapy (MCT) [3, 4, 5].

It is the only bacillus to multiply in the Schwann cells, also in the histiocytes and other cells such as muscle cells and vascular endothelium [6]. *M. leprae* still could not be cultivated '*in vitro*'. Such factor makes the study of its properties a difficult task. The incubation period is slow, from 2 to 7 years. It has high infectivity and low pathogenicity [7, 8], and the determinant factor for the manifestation or not of the disease is the immune status of the individual [9].

M. leprae was described in 1873 by a Norwegian, Gerhard Amauer Henrik Hansen. This discovery led to prompt rejection of the theory of hereditary transmission of this disease, which was supported by leading scholars of the 19th century. However, the acceptance that the infection and manifestations resulting from it depend largely on individual predisposition has still been the dominant paradigm [4].

Classification – Clinic – Reactions

Currently, the classification recommended by WHO for leprosy is based on the clinical presentation of the disease and on the lesion bacteriological index. According to number of lesions, the disease can be classified as: *single disease lesion* (01 lesion); *paucibacillary leprosy* - PB (02 - 05 skin lesions) ; and multibacillary leprosy- MB (more than 05 skin lesions) [2].

The PB operational form is represented by two clinical forms : *indeterminate form and tuberculoid form*. The MB operational form is also represented by two clinical forms: *borderline or dimorphic form and virchowian form* [10, 11] (Figure 1).

OPERATIONAL CLASSIFICATION (WHO)	SOLE LESION	PAUCIBACILLARY FEW BACILLI)	MULTIBACILLARY (MANY BACILLI)
CLINICAL FORMS	1-Undetermined 2- Tuberculoid	1- Undetermined 2- Tuberculoid	1-Dimorphi/Border-line 2-Virchowian

Source: WHO, 2010.

Figure 1. Operational Classification and Clinical Forms for Leprosy.

This method is easy to practical applicability; besides, it is reasonably balanced in terms of sensitivity and specificity, especially when compared to the classical division of Ridley and Jopling, 1966 [12] which presents 3 mixed clinical forms : *tuberculoid-dimorphic; dimorphic-dimorphic and virchowian-dimorphic* besides the *indeterminate, tuberculoid and virchowian forms*. Therefore, it is most used in research and takes into account the immunity within a spectrum of host resistance and the histopathology [2, 3, 11, 14, 15],

Another classification is the one from Madrid 1953, which considers two stable and opposite poles (*tuberculoid and Virchowian*) and two unstable poles (*Indeterminate and Dimorphic*) [16].

According to the classification of Jopling, there are two forms of leprosy reactions and they can occur before, during and after treatment. These are Type I and Type II reactions. In reaction Type I or Reversal Reaction (RR), cell immunity is impaired. Reaction Type II is clinically presented in the forms of Nodosum Erythema, Multiform Erythema or Necrotizing Erythema or 'Lucio's' Phenomenon, in which there is impairment of humoral immunity. These reactional states are present in 20-50 % of multibacillary cases and are considered risk factors for nerve lesions, causing disability and/or reinfection [17. 18].

The correct classification will lead to a more effective control of leprosy, by avoiding inadequate under or overtreatment and preventing recurrences [19].

The diagnosis is based on the clinical epidemiological examination (gold standard), and the following requisites must be observed: the presence of skin lesions with sensitivity alteration, and/or nerve involvement and/or positive bacilloscopy. Bacilloscopy was used as a reference for establishing sensitivity and specificity of the clinical criteria. Tests for thermal, painful and tactile sensitivities in the areas of lesions, bacilloscopy and histopathological examination are routinely used means as complimentary diagnosis [1].

Another diagnostic method such as Phenolic Glicolipid 1 (PGL-1) is also used. PGL-1 was described in 1998 as a specific immunogenic antigen of *M. leprae*. Thus, the first serological tests started to appear, and ELISA was the most commonly used for detecting antibodies against PGL-1 [9].

The ML-Flow was developed in 2003, and it is an immunocromatographic diagnostic test which detects IgM antibodies against the *M. leprae* PGL-1, by using blood. It is easy to perform and does not require specialized laboratory. The reagents are stable and can be stored at room temperature [19].

Treatment and Prophylactic Actions

Regarding treatment of pregnant or breastfeeding leprosy women, standard PQT treatment (rifampicin, clofazimine and dapsone) is not contraindicated at the recommended doses. Caution must be taken with the appearance of reactive states, especially the Type II ones, where thalidomide isthe first drug of choice, but due to its teratogenic potential is contraindicated during pregnancy and lactation period. However, other drugs may be prescribed, such as prednisone and/or acetyl salicylic acid and/or pentoxifylline. In Type I reaction, prednisone should still be the first choice. In cases of intolerance to any drug belonging to the PQT scheme, ofloxacin and/or minocycline may be the surrogate. As the neuritic pain, pregnant women may use antidepressants (amitriptyline and/or nortriptyline) and/or anticonvulsants (carbamazepine and/or gabapentin) [20].

A prophylactic action should be vaccination of contacts with BCG (Bacille Calmette Guerin). This vaccination is contraindicated during pregnancy and breastfeeding period [21, 2].

Surveillance of Leprosy

According to WHO in epidemiological statement issued in August 2010, more than 200,000 new cases were discovered in the world in 2009. Despite detection of new cases have been reduced annually between 2003 and 2009, rates of decline were mild compared to previous years from 2006 [2].

Worldwide, approximately 720,000 new cases of leprosy have been reported each year, and approximately two million people show disease sequels concerning this illness [10]. The six countries with the highest endemicity in the world in descending order: India, Brazil, Burma, Madagascar, Nepal and Mozambique. They account for 88 % of all new cases of leprosy in the world. Recent cohort studies have shown a peak of onset of this disease between 10 and 20 years old. After puberty, there are twice as many cases of leprosy in men than in women [10, 22].

The WHO considers the *detection Coeficient (Incidence and/or prevalence rate)* an important indicator no matter if it is detected for general leprosy, for leprosy associated with pregnancy[59] and also for youngsters under 15, the latter with much attention due to recent and active infection demonstration [21]. In Brazil, the term *'detection Coeficient'* is more commonly used than the term *'Incidence and/or prevalence rate'*. Skin lesions are considered the identifier signs of leprosy. These, when clinically examined accounts for the 'gold standard' diagnosis for the disease [24], although new techniques in molecular biology have already brought advances in the detection of specific nucleotide sequences of microorganisms [25]. A great part of the endemic regions classically present tropical climate with high temperatures and much rain [26]; although the disease had already shown high incidences in temperate and cold climates before being eradicated from those regions [27].

In the Americas, Brazil accounts for over 90% of reports, mainly at the expense of the northern region (Amazon), which has high rain index, equatorial climate and low socio - economic level. All in all these facts account for the high incidence of both general leprosy and its association with pregnancy. This adverse association between low socio economic and cultural level, plus the presence of sequels, demonstrates the vulnerability of this population and incur loss of quality of life, because current treatment options do not include additional reversibility to the leprosy stigma [14, 28]. Leprosy is a socially produced aggravation. Therefore, it is very complex for a simple elimination paradigm [23. 29].

Strategies such as 'elimination plans' and 'control plans' have been employed especially in endemic countries with the purpose of achieving the goal that is determinated by WHO to eliminate leprosy as a public health problem by 2015, with less than a case per 10,000 inhabitants [2].

The control is based on early diagnosis of cases, effective treatment for healing, identification of the source of infection and risk factors, aiming at avoiding the evolution of the injury to usually irreversible nerve damage, which causes deformities as sequels, creating limitations and functional disability [1].

The operation for the control of a disease depends on detailed and accurate information in order to support planning, design of strategies and resource targeting [30].

Evidence concerning the importance of genetic factors [31], as well as cultural - socio -economic illness such as children and elderly patients with severe multibacillary forms of the disease living together in small rooms which are occupied by many people. This reality impels the need of even more focus on the importance of surveillance and even prophylaxis of these people who are in contact with those known index-cases of leprosy [32, 33, 34, 35].

Epidemiological surveillance of leprosy involves collection, processing, analysis and interpretation of data from patients and their contacts aiming at: case detection, early treatment, skin and neurological examinations for all contacts. The correct diagnosis of leprosy requires understanding the spectral concept of it, so there is a correlation between the clinical course of the disease and the extent of the neural damage in accordance with the characteristic of each clinical form [24].

The strategy of eliminating leprosy may be regarded as most remarkable and controversial in leprosy control since the adoption of compulsory isolation of cases. There are those who consider it highly positive and those who are against its implementation. Both groups have remarkable evidences to support their positions [36, 37]. However, the adoption of PCT seems to be a common ground of agreement between the groups. In fact, the MDT is a key element for the treatment of leprosy in any strategy because of its efficiency and also because monotherapy with dapsone or any other anti-leprosy drug should be regarded as unethical practice [38].

The detection rates and the lack of an effective vaccine to prevent the disease indicate that leprosy will continue to be an important public health problem in many countries, and for several decades. Thus, it should be understood that the period of leprosy elimination strategy had its time and its relevance mainly by the enormous political support caused by the gravity of the disease. However, the lessons learned by the implementation of these strategies clearly indicate that new approaches should be thought and discussed to tackle such disease that, despite the outstanding reduction in prevalence, it continues to be present in major countries of the world like India and Brazil [39].

Thus, emphasis should be given as a preliminary approach to the continuity of basic and operational research, because many questions still need to be answered not only with regard to the understanding of the disease transmission, chain and treatment, but also with the relating mechanism between mycobacteria and Schwann cells so that they do not reach to cause nerve damage. Thus, by fulfilling the 'elimination' step as a strategy, new contribution must be given by health authorities and researchers regarding these questions, which include, hereby, continuing support for research and training of human resources in leprosy [40, 41].

Leprosy and Pregnancy

Leprosy and pregnancy occurring together constitute an association between an infectious and contagious disease and a particular physiological state of a restricted populational fragment: women. The association between leprosy and pregnancy is uncommon, unlike the complications that can come with such a relationship [42].

The hormonal, metabolic and immunologic changes due to pregnancy generally reflect low immunity in this period and let women more vulnerable to diseases, especially infectocontagious ones. Therefore, the appearance of type I or type II reactional states of leprosy is not uncommon, due to the onset of clinical leprosy during pregnancy [21].

The pregnancy period has been strongly related to the appearance and worsening of clinical symptoms of leprosy mainly between the last trimester of pregnancy and the first three months of lactation (postpartum), probably due to the inherent typical changes during pregnancy. During the last pregnancy trimester, there is relatively depression in cellular immunity, with worsening of Type II leprosy reactions. There may be the appearance of a typical reactive form known as 'Lúcio's Phenomenon or Reaction', which added to the typical pregnancy vascular changes, result in a truly serious situation of necrotizing vasculitis. During postpartum, there is suppression of humoral immunity with enhancement of Type I reactions. These have quick installation and result in nerve damage, causing necrosis. Some researchers mistakenly call it 'nerve abscess', but they cause irreversible damages [43, 44].

Leprosy in pregnancy should be worrisome for the surveillance agencies, because the chosen drug for treatment when reactional type II episodes occur is thalidomide, known as teratogenic [45].

The 'Lúcio's phenomenon' is characterized by necrotic lesions of nodosum or polymorphic erythema during the evolution of a framework for leprosy in patients with or without lepromas [43].

The lack of more detailed studies on the general contemporary aspects of leprosy associated with pregnancy studies is evident. The few studies with this approach are almost entirely sponsored by the surveillance and health promotion governmental institutions, but the scientific nongovernmental initiative is more dedicated to more specific correlated themes. The serious problems responsible for the difficulty in adapting the statistics to the aims at elimination of leprosy within the deadlines set by the WHO, such as late diagnosis, non- adherence to treatment by patients and failures in the flow of registration and notification require further clarification to enable the review strategies and the adoption of new measures to eliminate general leprosy as a public health problem, which promotes unwavering character for exposure and analysis of the factors that make up the actual current leprosy situation in relation to the period of pregnancy [2, 46].

Some of the common laboratory abnormalities in pregnant women affected by leprosy are: mild anemia, mild leukocytosis with a left shift and when bacilloscopy is positive, it generally shows high bacilli index, which predicts operational MB form [43, 42]. Some non-specific serological tests like VDRL (about 40 % of cases) and specific as FTA-ABS (about 16 %) for syphilis may be false-positive by cross reaction with leprosy [42].

In some studies, about 50% of pregnant patients with leprosy have obstetric complications. These mostly occur in multibacillary forms. There are reports of increased incidence of ectopic pregnancy, fetal death and prematurity [42]. Newborns from leprosy mothers have lower birth weight and have a higher incidence of respiratory problems due to placental insufficiency and slow intrauterine growth [43].

No later than sixty years ago, Ryrie wrote: 'within the interaction between pregnancy and associated pathological conditions, leprosy seems to be one of the few systemic diseases in which such action is entirely one-sided. Leprosy seems to have no effect on pregnancy, but pregnancy has a marked effect on the course of leprosy'. Leprosy showed no effect on the first menstruation, menstrual cycle or fertility, as opposed to men in that sterility can occur after engagement of the bacillum with the testicles [47].

Regarding immunological issues of pregnancy in leprosy, there is relatively suppressed activity of T-cells (T-lymphocytes) during pregnancy. Thus pregnant women are more susceptible to infections such as hepatitis and intracellular pathogens such as toxoplasmosis. Thus, pregnancy could also lead to increased risk for the development of diseases including leprosy. Case reports of the last sixty years have documented either the relationship between pregnancy and the first diagnosis of leprosy or an exacerbation of symptoms in patients with the disease already established [47], and even the reactivation of lesions in previously treated and presumably cured patients. Some studies, such as Rodriguez et al. (2009) report such worsening of disease activity during pregnancy in patients with leprosy [48].

The increased activity of leprosy during pregnancy may be due to either the disease progression or to immunological complications. It has already been reported the so-called ‘aggravation of leprosy during pregnancy’. However, it has not been clear of what the term ‘aggravation’ would be. Therefore. it is unclear, however, whether the reference is to the progression of the disease or to the appearance of reactive states [47].

A theory of immunological complications during pregnancy says part of pregnancy physiology occurs with relatively suppressed maternal immune response, thus being directed away from the cell-mediated immunity towards humoral immunity. There is a negative regulation of type Th1 (T helper 1 limphocytes) answer during pregnancy with decreased production of IL-2 (interleukin 2), especially during the third trimester of pregnancy [47].

Seventeen percent of women with rheumatoid arthritis (an autoimmune disease mediated by cells) experience a temporary remission of their symptoms during pregnancy, therefore considered as a protective factor. In contrast, systemic erythematosus lupus (an also autoimmune disease, but antibody-mediated), worsens during pregnancy. In this case, it is considered a risk factor. Thus, it can be inferred that the type 1 leprosy whose reactions are due to enhanced cellular immunity against *M. leprae*, would be improved during pregnancy, whereas type 2 leprosy (Nodosum erythema Leprosy), which occur mainly due to deposit of immune complexes and complement activation, would be increased during the pregnancy period [47].

In a prospective cohort study in Ethiopia, reactions were reported in all trimesters of pregnancy. However, this data analysis becomes impossible in the absence of control, which was a consequence of the lack of methodological rigor in those days [49].

One theory about the stages of puerperium and lactation, claims that there is a recovery of cellular immunity in the mother immediately after birth, and this issue sets women at risk for immune-mediated complications. Although puerperium and breastfeeding are well recognized by ancient leprosy researchers as a period in which acute reactions may occur, it was only in 1975 that the first series of cases of pregnancy-associated reactions has been published [50].

Duncan and Pearson’s data show a clear association between puerperium and the development of neuritis. Patients have been reported with evident neuritis, i.e., pain and/or nerve sensitivity, and also patients with silent neuritis, that is, with sensory and/or motor decreased function with neither pain nor nerve sensibility. The association between neuritis and postpartum was stronger in patients with dimorphic and virchowan clinical forms [50].

Few obstetric problems have been reported in women with leprosy, regardless of the type of disease. Duncan found uncomplicated pregnancies in Ethiopia. However, in a cohort study, infants of leprosy mothers weighed significantly less than those of other mothers without leprosy. Also estrogen excretion test was performed in these studies (as an index of fetoplacental function), and the result of the uteroplacental perfusion was decreased [50].

The repercussions of leprosy surpasses the boundaries of health institutions, since their relationship with the occurrence of deformities and consequent disability entails abstinence from work, need for specialized technical resources and hence economic burden. Furthermore, cultural stigma of sin and God punishment related to leprosy creep from biblical times to the present days, leading to social segregation and loss of quality of life [51].

The frequent association between Hansen's disease and social illnesses and the need for data on the disease require a reinterpretation of current epidemiological indicators which donot depict situations of collective risks that can explain how this disease produces itself socially.

The study of the interaction profile between leprosy and pregnancy status becomes extremely necessary. On the one hand, if leprosy commonly does not bring serious repercussions on pregnancy; pregnancy, with its immunological, metabolic and hormonal alterations, can dramatically change the course of a leprosy framework [51].

Through the State University of Pará and the Evandro Chagas Institute (Amazon, Brazil) research group, Palácios et al. (2011) created a new epidemiological indicator: the so cal*led 'Coefficient for Detection of Leprosy linked to Pregnancy'(CDLP)* or *'Rate for Prevalence and/or Incidence of leprosy associated to Pregnancy'*, byshowing the new interpretation parameters for this indicator whenever leprosy is associated with pregnancy. In order to perform the epidemiological analysis, top-down and botton-up methods were used by considering the many social, economical and demographic territorial features and their fragments. This indicator allows incidence, prevalence, trend studies. In Brazil, northeastern and northern regions are the ones with the greatest CDLP [23, 52, 60] (Figure 2).

PARAMETERS (PER 10,000 INHABITANTS)	GENERAL LEPROSY*	LEPROSY IN CHILDREN UNDER 15 YEARS OF AGE*	LEPROSY ASSOCIATED TO PREGNANCY**
HIPERENDEMIC	Equal or higher than 4 cases	Equal or higher than 1 case	Equal or higher than 2 cases
VERY HIGH	2 to 3.9 cases	0.5 a 0.99 cases	1.35 to 1.99 cases
HIGH	1 to 1.99 cases	0.25 a 0.49 cases	0.75 to 1.34 cases
AVERAGE	0.2 to 0.9 cases	0.05 a 0.24 cases	0.45 to 0.74 cases
LOW	Lower than 0.2 cases	Lower than 0.05 cases	Lower than 0.45 cases

Source: WHO, 2005 *. Source: Palácios et al., 2011. **

Figure 2. Prevalence Rates. Interpretation of endemicity parameters for general leprosy; for children under 15; for association between leprosy and pregnancy.

For the CDLP Calculus: the numerator is represented by the total number of pregnant leprosy women and, as denominator, the total number of women aged 12 to 49 years (selected age range which corresponds to fertile age), multiplied by 10,000 or 100,000 inhabitants, depending on quantitative population for adequacy of analysis [23, 60].

$$\text{CDLP} = \frac{\text{n° of pregnants leprosy women}}{\text{Total n° of women aged } 12 - 49} \text{ x } 10{,}000$$

It required the creation of CDLP indicator for the analysis of leprosy epidemiological situation when associated with pregnancy so that qualitative and quantitative analysis could be generated. The CDLP permitted to assess the epidemiological scenario of this biological interaction initially in Brazil, thus serving as a new and useful tool for planning and adopting measures of surveillance and control of the fearsome consequences of coexistence between the disease caused by M. leprae and the formation process of a new human being [43, 47, 49, 50, 52].

According to Veiga (2005), the analysis in health context incorporates technologies from other areas of knowledge such as geoprocessing, which is applied on environmental and socioeconomic issues. According to WHO, the identification of *cluster* corridors of leprosy corridors serves to monitor the behavior of the disease and the indication areas of greatest risk of transmission and show where the majority of cases are located [52].

The implantation of developmental projects such as mining, hydroelectric, lumber, industry, agriculture and crop sectors, and unplanned urbanization create factors that make up an epidemiological setting conducive to the emergence and growth of diseases, especially infectious contagious ones, like leprosy. This scenery, in underdeveloped countries, favor the settlement of human conglomerates and the formation of poverty belts. As a consequence, malnutrition, lack of adequate living conditions as poor sanitation, difficulties with housing, promiscuity, clothing, pregnancies without proper planning and other ills that are determinant factors of diseases [20, 53, 54].

The interpersonal contact promoted by professional activities is a major factor for spreading leprosy, and this shall also be related to the occurrence of leprosy associated with pregnancy, prevention and control and the same argument applies to their association [15, 53].

Nerve injury is associated with physical disability and deformity. It is considered the most severe complication of leprosy. Therefore, it is obvious that there is a clear need for this to be part of prenatal care program. Thus, all pregnant women should be referred to the dermatological examination, which is a simple procedure, because it is only a visual examination (inspection). This so simple and so effective procedure does not make part of the prenatal program for the control of pregnant women in underdeveloped and developing countries such as India and Brazil. This matter confirms the negligence of the surveillance services. The lack of such procedures allow and perpetuate serious complications during pregnancy which could be avoided or minimized. Thus, favoring the maintenance of the endemicity [15].

Ferreira et al., demonstrated that the presence of more than five household contacts double the risk of relapses in general leprosy. According to Santos et al[57] the risk of developing the disease is 5-10 times higher if a family member has already expressed leprosy. Moreover, it is necessary to conduct periodic examinations of contacts, because only a small number of cases is detected at the moment the index case was diagnosed [56].

Leprosy, its social burden, and its complex and multifaceted epidemiological environment make up a real blight on public health and, when combined with a physiological condition as odd as pregnancy, it becomes a labyrinth for those who are dedicated to their study. Also, the large gap in recent decades as to technical and scientific work on such associations makes up for a practically nil existence of updated theoretical framework and methodological quality studies. Thus, the creation of an indicator for the interpretation of new parameter for the association of endemicity of leprosy and pregnancy, became necessary for examination of the epidemiological situation. According to CDLP, not only the behavior of this disease when associated with pregnancy, but also the general leprosy, itself, has been falling down each year in most still endemic countries, although slowly [40, 58].

References

[1] Grossi, M.A.F.; Lebaeuf, M.A.A.; Andrade, A.R.C.; Lyon,S.; Antunes,C.M.F.; Bührer-Sékula,S. A influência do teste sorológico ML Flow na classificação da hanseníase. *Rev. Soc. Bras. Med. Trop.,* 41(suplemento II): 34-38, 2008.

[2] World Health Organization. Weekly epidemiological record – 27 august 2010. Geneva: *Who,* 2010. p. 337-348.

[3] Sampaio, S.A.P.; Rivitti, E.A.; Marchese, L.M.T. Hanseníase. In: Sampaio, S.A.P.; Rivitti, E.A. Dermatologia. 2. ed. São Paulo: Artes Médicas, 2010. p. 467-488.

[4] Beiguelman, B. Genética e hanseníase. Ciênc. Saúde Coletiva. v. 7, n. 1, p. 117-128, 2002.

[5] Jopling, W.H.; Mcdougall, A.C. Manual de Hanseníase. 4. ed. São Paulo, 1991.

[6] Ribeiro, S.L.E.; Guedes, E.L.; Pereira, H.L.A.; Souza, L.S. Vasculite na hanseníase mimetizando doenças reumáticas. *Rev. Bras. Reumatol.,* v. 47, n. 2, p. 140-144, mar-abr. 2007.

[7] Nishino, L. Hanseníase – alterações imunológicas, 1997. Disponível em: <http://www.saudetotal.com/artigos/diversos/hanseníase.asp>. Acesso em: 27 out. 2007, 15:56:34.

[8] Goulart, I.M.B.; Penna, G.O.; Cunha, G. Imunopatologia da hanseníase: a complexidade dos mecanismos de respostas imune do hospedeiro ao Mycobacterium leprae. *Rev. Soc. Bras. Med. Trop.,* v. 35, n. 4, p. 365-375, jul-ago. 2002.

[9] Maeda, Y. et al. Identification of an immunomodulation agent from *Mycobacterium leprae.* Infect. Immun., v. 73, n. 7, p. 4458, jul. 2005.

[10] Lockwood, D. Leprosy. BMJ, 2007. Disponível em: <http://clinicalevidence.bmj.com/ceweb/conditions/ind/0915/0915_backgr.jsp>. Acesso em: 15 set. 2010, 16:17:09.

[11] Croft, R.P.; Smith, W.C.S.; Nicholls, P; Richardus, J.H. Sensitivity and specificity of methods of classification of leprosy without use of skin-smear examination. *Int. J. Lepr. Other Mycobact. Dis.,* dez. 1998.

Disponível em: <http://findarticles.com/p/articles/mi_qa3754/is_199812 /ai_n8814503>. Acesso em: 12 set. 2010, 12:23:45.

[12] Ridlei,D.S.; Jopling,W.H. Classification of leprosy according to immunity: a five group systen. *International Journal of Leprosy and Other Mycrobacterial Diseases,* 34:255-273, 1996.

[13] AvelleiRA, J.C. et al. Micobacterioses. In: AzULAY, R.D.; AzuLAY, D.R. Dermatologia. 3. ed. Rio de Janeiro: Guanabara Koogan, 2004. p. 223-233.

[14] Burdick, A.E.; Capó, V.A.; Frankel, S. Micobacteria. In: Tyring, S.K.; Lupi, O; Hengge, U.R. Tropical Dermatology. 1. ed. Philadelphia: Elsevier Churchill Livingstone, 2006. p. 255-271.

[15] Moschioni, C.; Antunes, C.M.F.; Grossi, M.A.F.; Lambertucci, J.R. Risk factors for physical disability at diagnosis of 19,283 new cases of leprosy. Rev. Soc. Bras. Med. Trop., v. 43, n. 1, p. 19-22, jan-fev. 2010.

[16] Araújo, M.G. Hanseníase no Brasil. *Rev. Soc. Bras. Med. Trop.,* v. 36, n. 3, p. 373-382, mai-jun. 2003.

[17] Teixeira, M.A.G.; Silveira, V.M.; França, E.R. Características epidemiológicas e clínicas das reações hansênicas em indivíduos paucibacilares e multibacilares atendidos em dois centros de referência para hanseníase, na cidade de Recife, Estado de Pernambuco. *Rev. Soc. Bras. Med. Trop.,* v. 43, n. 3, p. 287-292, mai-jun. 2010.

[18] Brasil. Ministério da Saúde. Departamento de Informática do SUS. Portal da Saúde. Situação epidemiológica da hanseníase. MS, 2007. Disponível em: <http://www.saude.gov.br/portal/arquivos/pdf/situação_ hansen_2007.pdf>. Acesso em: 12 set. 2010, 15:44:44.

[19] Büther-Sékula; Smitis,H.L.; Gussenhaven,G.C.; Leeuwen,J.; Amador,S.; Fujiwara, T.; Klatser,P.R.; OscAN,L. Simple and fast lateral flow test for classification of leprosy patients and identification of contats with high risk of developing leprosy. *Journal of Clinical Microbiology,* 41: 1991-1995, 2003.

[20] Brasil. Secretaria de Vigilância em Saúde. Situação da hanseníase no Brasil. 2008. Informe epidemiológico. Disponível em: <http://www. saude.gov.br/svs>. Acesso em: 28 fev. 2011, 14:14:14.

[21] BrASIL. Ministério da Saúde. Secretaria de Vigilância em Saúde. Plano Nacional de Eliminação da Hanseníase. V carta de eliminação da hanseníase-Pará. Brasil: MS, 2006. p. 01-02.

[22] World Health Organization. Guide to eliminate leprosy as a public health problem. Geneva: WHO. 2006.

[23] Palácios, V.R.C.M.; Bichara, C.N.C.; Dias, R.S.; Fontelles, M.J.P.; Veiga, N.G. Leprosy and pregnancy in the state of Pará:an epidemiological perspective. *Rev Sos. Bras. Med. Trop.,* Jul-Ago, 2013.

[24] Xavier, M.B.; Cunha, M.H.C.M.; Macedo, G.M.M.; Batista, K.N.M.; Neto, S.S.; Nascimento, F.S.N. Avaliação clinico-epidemiológica em pacientes multibacilares em uma unidade de referência em hansenologia da Amazônia. Hansen. Int., v. 33, n. 2, p. 09-16, 2008.

[25] Assis, N.C.S.; Lopes, M.L.; Cardoso, N.C.; Costa, M.M.; Sousa, C.O.; Lima, K.V.B. Diagnóstico molecular da tuberculose pulmonar. *J. Bras. Patol. Med. Lab.,* v. 43, n. 1, p. 1-7, fev. 2007.

[26] Magalhães, M.M.C.; Rojas, L.I. Diferenciação territorial da hanseníase no Brasil. Epidemiol. Serv. Saúde, v. 16, n. 2, p. 75-84, abr-jun. 2007.

[27] Meima, A.; Irgens, L.M.; Oortmarssen, G.J.V.; Richardus, J.A.; Habbema, J.D.F. Disappearance of leprosy from Norway: an exploration of critical factors using an epidemiological modelling approach. *Int. J. Epidemiol.,* v. 31, n. 5, p. 991-1000, out. 2002.

[28] Duarte, E.C. et al. Epidemiologia das desigualdades em saúde no Brasil: um estudo exploratório. Brasília: OPAS, 2002 apud Magalhães, M.C.C.; Rojas, L.I. Epidemiol. Serv. Saúde, v. 16, n. 2, p. 75-84, abr-jun. 2007.

[29] Loockwood,D.N.J.; Suneethas. Leprosy: too complex a disease for a simple elimination paradigm. *Bull World Health Organ,* Geneve. V.83: p.230-235, 2005.

[30] Galvão, P.R.S. et al. Uma avaliação do sistema de informação SinAN usado no Programa de Controle de Hanseníase no estado do Pernambuco, Brasil. Cad. Saúde Colet., v. 17, n. 1, p. 87-102, 2009.

[31] Durães, S.M.B.; Guedes, L.S.; Cunha, M.D.; Cavaliere, F.A.M.; Oliveira, M.L.W.D.R. Estudo de 20 focos familiars de hanseníase no município de Duque de Caxias, Rio de Janeiro. An. Bras. Dermatol., v.80, n.supl3, p. s295-300, nov-dez. 2005.

[32] Oliveira, B.F.A.; Ignotti, E.; Hartwuig, S.V.; Scatena, J.H.; Andrade, V.L.G. Acréscimo na detecção de casos de hanseníase como resultado da vigilância de comunicantes em 15 municípios considerados prioritários do estado do Mato Grosso, Brasil. Espaç. saúde, v. 8, n. 2, p. 11-19, jun. 2007.

[33] Nery, J.A.; Bernardes, F.F.; Quintanilha, J.; Machado, A.M.; Oliveira, S.S.; Sales, A.M. Understanding the type I reacional state for early diagnosis and tratment: a way to avoid disability in leprosy. *An Bras. Dermatol.,* Sep-Oct.88(5):787-792, 2013.

[34] Sanches, L.A.T.; Pittner, E.; Sanches, H.F.; Monteiro, M.C. Detecção de casos novos de hanseníase no município de Prudentópolis, PR: Uma análise de 1998 a 2005. *Rev. Soc. Bras. Med.,* Trop., v. 40, n. 5, p. 541-545, out. 2007.

[35] Andrade, V. New approach to accelerate the elimination of leprosy. *Hansen. Int. Bauru,* v.24, n., p. 49-54,1994.

[36] Dogra, S.; Nran, T.; Kumar, B. Leprosy- evolution of the path to erradication. *Indian J. Med. Res.,* Mumbai, v.37,p.15-35,2013.

[37] FinE,P. Leprosy: what is being eliminated? *Bull. World Health Organ.,* Geneva, v.85, n.1,p.2,2007.

[38] GloBAL situation of leprosy control at the beginning of the 21st century. Lep Rev. London, v.73, s,p.15-16,2012.

[39] Sunda Rao Pss. Worldwide Elimination of Leprosy. *Expert Rev. Dermatol.,* London, v.7, n.6,p. 513-520,2012.

[40] WHO. Leprosy today. Available at: http://www.who.int/lep/en /2012

[41] Marcano, G.; González, M.E.; Vidal, J.; Moreno, C.; Zamora, A. Enfermedad de Hansen y Embarazo a Proposito de Dos Casos. Dermatologia Venezolana, v. 31, n. 3, p. 105-108, 1993.

[42] Helmer, K.A.; Fleischfresser, I.; Esmanhoto, L.D.K.; Neto, J.F.; Santamaria, J.R. Fenômeno de Lúcio (Eritema necrosante) na gestação. *An. Bras. Dermatol.,* v. 79, n. 2, p. 205-210, mar-abr. 2004.

[43] Rodríguez-Pazos, L.; Gómez-Bernal, S.; Sánchez-Aguilar, D.; TORIBIO, J. Lepra reaction and pregnancy. Actas Dermosifiliogr., v. 101, n. 2, p. 190-191, 2010.

[44] Brasil. Ministério da Saúde. Secretaria de Vigilância em Saúde. Departamento de Vigilância Epidemiológica. Programa Nacional de Eliminação da Hanseníase. Hanseníase. In: Guia de Vigilância Epidemiológica. 7. ed. Brasília: MS, 2009. cad. 7. p. 1-28.

[45] Cunha, M.D. et al. Os indicadores da hanseníase e as estratégias de eliminação da doença em município endêmico do estado do Rio de Janeiro, Brasil. Cad. Saúde Pública, v. 23, n. 5, p. 1187-1197, mai. 2007.

[46] Lockwood, D.N.G.; Sinha, H.H. Pregnancy and leprosy: a comprehensive leterature review. *Int. J. Lepr. Other Mycobact. Dis.,* v. 67, n. 1, p. 6-12, mar. 1999.

[47] Trindade, M.A.B.; Valente, N.Y.S.; Manini, M.I.P.; Takahashi, M.D.F.; Anjos, C.F.D.; Bernard, G.; Naafs, B. Two Patients Coinfected with Mycobacterium leprae and Human Immunodeficiency Virus Type 1 and NaÏve for Antiretroviral Therapy Who Exhibited Type 1 Leprosy

Reactions Mimicking the Immune Reconstitution Inflammatory Syndrome. *J. Clin. Microbiol.,* v. 44, n. 12, p. 4616-4618, 2006.

[48] DuncAN, M. E. An historical and clinical review of the interaction of leprosy and pregnancy: a cycle to be broken, s. 1, s. n, p. 1-16, 1993

[49] Duncan, M.E.; Oakey, R.E. Estrogen excretion in pregnant women with leprosy: evidence of diminished fetoplacental function, s. 1, s. n, p. 1-5, jul. 1982.

[50] BrasiL. Ministério da Saúde. Secretaria de Vigilância em Saúde. Departamento de Vigilância Epidemiológica. Programa Nacional de Controle da Hanseníase. Indicadores de monitoramento e comportamento da hanseníase no Brasil. Brasília: MS, 2008.

[51] Veiga, N.G. Modelo de Estruturação do Banco Georreferenciado de dados Ambientais, Epidemiológicos e Socioeconômico de Bragança-Pa. Belém: IECSVS/MS. Relatório Técnico, 2005.

[52] World Heath OrganizatION. Leprosy today. WHO, 2007. Disponível em: <http://www.who.int/lep/en/>. Acesso em: 15 set. 2010, 12:12:12.

[53] Penna,M.L.; Penna, G. O. Trand of case detection and leprosy elimination in Brazil. Trop. Med. Int. Health, Oxford, v.12, n.5, p. 647-650, 2007.

[54] Palácios, V.R.C.M.; Neves, D.C.O. Estudo da Situação da Hanseníase no Estado do Pará. *Rev. Para. Med.,* v. 24, n. 2, p. 49-56, abr-jun, 2010.

[55] Ferreira, S.M.B.; Ignotti, E.; Gamba, M.A. Fatores associados à recidiva em hanseníase em Mato Grosso. Rev. Saúde Pública, v. 45, n. 4, p. 756-764, jul-ago. 2011.

[56] Santos, A.S.; Castro, D.S.; Falqueto, A. Fatores de risco para transmissão da Hanseníase. Rev. Bras. Enferm., v. 61, n. Esp, p. 738-743. 2008.

[57] Brasil. Ministério da Saúde. Departamento de Informática do SUS. Portal da Saúde. Hanseníase - Casos confirmados notificados no Sistema de Informação de Agravos de Notificação - Sinan Net. 2011. Disponível em: <http://dtr2004.saude.gov.br/sinanweb/tabnet/dh?sinannet/hanseniase/bases/Hansbrnet.def>. Acesso em: 15 fev. 2012, 10:10:10.

[58] Palácios, V.R.C.M.; Bichara, C.N.C.; Andriolo, R.B.; Fontelles, M.J.P.; VEIGA, N.G.Analysis of the detection coefficient, for the association between leprosy and pregnancy in the region of Carajas, state of Pará, Brasil. *Rev Sos. Bras. Med.,* Trop. Jul-Ago, 2013.

[59] Palácios, V.R.C.M.; Bichara, C.N.C.; Andriolo, R.B.; Fontelles, M.J.P.; VEIGA, N.G. Analysis of the detection coefficient, for the association

between leprosy and pregnancy in the region of Carajas, state of Pará, Brasil. *Rev. Sos. Bras. Med. Trop.,* Jul-Ago, 2013.

[60] Palácios Palácios, V.R.C.M.; Bichara, C.N.C.; Andriolo, R.B.; Fontelles, M.J.P.; Veiga, N.G. Póvoa,M.M. Leprosy and pregnancy: detection coefficient, proposal a new index. *Rev. Sos. Bras. Med. Trop.,* Admitted to publication in may-20-2014.

In: Leprosy
Editor: Roger S. Kopp

ISBN: 978-1-63321-668-6

Chapter 4

The Potential of Antimicrobial Peptide Inhibitors (APIs) and Elicitors (APEs) in Leprosy Treatment

Ernesto Prado Montes de Oca[1,2,*]
[1]*In silico* laboratory
[2]Molecular Biology Laboratory, Biosafety Area, Medical and Pharmaceutical Biotechnology Unit, Research Center in Technology and Design Assistance of Jalisco State, National Council of Science and Technology (CIATEJ AC, CONACYT), Guadalajara, México

Abstract

Antimicrobial peptides or host defense peptides as defensins and hepcidin are fundamental components of human innate immunity. A growing body of recent evidence suggests they have a role in a broad range of diseases as cancer, allergies and infections, including leprosy.

---

* Corresponding author: Ernesto Prado Montes de Oca. 1) In silico laboratory, 2) Molecular Biology Laboratory, Biosafety Area, Medical and Pharmaceutical Biotechnology Unit, Research Center in Technology and Design Assistance of Jalisco State, National Council of Science and Technology (CIATEJ AC, CONACYT), Guadalajara, México. E-mail: eprado @ciatej.mx.

Antimicrobial peptide inhibitors (APIs) are physical, chemical or biological agents that downregulate human antimicrobial peptide expression. In leprosy there is upregulation of both hepcidin and human beta defensin 3 which leads to opportunities for intervention.

In the case of the hepcidin-mediated iron sequestration, this can enhance opportunistic infections and a possible role in facilitating *Mycobacterium leprae* growth. Corticosteroid prednisolone suppresses human beta-defensins 2 and 3 in leprosy patients with type 1 reactions (T1R). However, costicosteroids inhibits the NF-κB pathway that causes immune suppression in the long term. These reactions are the main cause of nerve damage in leprosy.

Additionally, antimicrobial peptide elicitors (APEs) of human beta defensins could help to enhance the antimycobacterial response against *M. leprae*. The challenge is to find specific and mild inhibitors as APIs that combat T_H1 inflammatory response without compromising the host immune system or use in combination with APEs of defensins. In this context, APIs and APEs could help in leprosy treatment with lessened induction to side effects. This could be helpful as a new and/or adjunctive therapy to find novel and specific APIs, APEs and/or anti-inflammatory agents in order to limit *M. leprae* growth and prevent nerve damage in leprosy patients.

Introduction

Leprosy (or Hansen disease) is a chronic granulomatous infectious disease caused by the obligate intracellular organism *Mycobacterium leprae* [1]. Due to the lipid content of the cell wall, *M. leprae* infection can leave behind persistent antigens within affected skin and nerve tissues making patients vulnerable to unpredictable leprosy reactions years after they are clinical cured. Type 1 reactions (T1Rs or reversal reactions) represent the acute immune episodes of T_H1 inflammatory response to *M. leprae* antigens. These reactions occur in the skin and/or nerves and are the leading causes of neurological impairment in leprosy patients [1]. Peripheral nerve damage is an important issue in clinical leprosy, a complication that diminishes patient´s quality of life. In lepromatous leprosy (L-lep), the most severe and disseminated form of the disease, nerve function impairment occurs earlier than in tuberculoid leprosy, the localized and mild form of the disease. The destruction of dermal nerves mainly affects hands, feet and legs (this pattern is often referred as “glove and stocking” neuropathy), peripheral nerve damage occurs late.

Also, there is bacterial proliferation within the Schwann cells, which leads to foamy degeneration of the cells losing their regeneration ability.

This nerve damage causes deformities and disabilities as well as social stigma and discrimination of patients and their families. The T1R are commonly treated with oral corticosteroids as prednisolone. However, costicosteroids commonly inhibit the NF-κB pathway that causes immune suppression in the long term including the downregulation of hBD-2 and cathelicidin LL-37. In addition to its direct antimicrobial activity, hBD-2 induces cytokines including IL-10, IL-8 and IL-6 in monocytes [2]. During TIRs, hBD3 is significantly upregulated in the skin. Also, keratinocytes but not macrophages upregulate hBD2 and hBD3 in response to *M. leprae in vitro* [2].

Anemia and hypoxia, two conditions related to oxygen availability, decrease the production of hepcidin, a small cationic liver-derived antimicrobial peptide that is a master regulator of iron metabolism causing degradation of ferroportin [3]. Hepcidin is present primarily in multibacillary (MB) lesions. It has been suggested that hepcidin-mediated iron sequestration could promote *M. leprae* growth [2]. Antimicrobial peptide inhibitors (APIs) of hepcidin could help in leprosy treatment with lessened induction to side effects. This could be helpful as a new and/or adjunctive therapy to find novel and specific APIs and/or anti-inflammatory agents in order to limit *M. leprae* growth and prevent nerve damage in leprosy patients.

Side Effects in the Traditional Treatment of Leprosy

Even when leprosy can be cured with available treatment, many of the antileprotic approved drugs cause side effects and drug resistance. Furthermore, even though there are methods to detect drug resistance-determining regions (DRDRs) in *M. leprae*, that could diminish the burden and cost of the disease, they are not widely applied in public health [4, 5].

Multi-drug therapy (MDT) for leprosy is currently comprised of clofazimine, dapsone, and rifampicin [6]. With regard to gender effects, females (OR=2.36) are less tolerant to multi-drug therapy than males as suggested in a report of the Brazilian population [7]. Results suggest that MDT can reduce the antioxidant activity of some enzymes and influence reactive oxygen species (ROS) accumulation, which may induce hematological changes, such as methemoglobinemia in patients with leprosy [8].

Clofazimine, a fat-soluble dye, has been used for leprosy since the 1960´s [9]. In a Brazilian sample population, clofazimine administered alone induced 21.6 % of the side effects (mainly reddish skin pigmentation) [10]. Another drawback of clofazimine is that it can cause crystal-storing histiocitosis and gastrointestinal disorders, sometimes with severe abdominal pain [11].

Dapsone (diamino-diphenyl sulfone) has been widely used in leprosy and several chronic inflammatory dermatological conditions. Dapsone is not a typical non-steroidal anti-inflammatory drug (NSAID) because it does not block cyclo-oxygenases. Dapsone instead inhibits bacterial synthesis of dihydrofolic acid via competition with para-aminobenzoate for the active site of dihydropteroate synthetase. However, its use induces hypersensitivity (1.4% of cases) that are sometimes fatal (in 9.9% of the reactions) [12].

Dapsone is known to cause hemolytic anemia (HA) and it seems this occurs more frequently than reported. In a Brazilian sample population, HA was present in 24.7% of the patients and occurs within the first 3 months in 51% of these cases [6]. Host genetic susceptibility also was demonstrated as relevant because allele HLA-B*13:01 is associated with the dapsone hypersensitivity syndrome (OR= 20.53) [13].

Rifamycins are a member of the ansamycin family of antibiotics. Rifamycin was extracted from fermentation cultures of *Amycolatopsis rifamycinica* (formerly *Streptomyces mediterranei*). It actually consisted of seven substances and therefore was renamed rifamycin A, B, C, D, E, S and SV. Rifamycin B is the most stable, least toxic, and active against a broad spectrum of bacteria, mainly Gram-positive cocci and *Mycobacterium tuberculosis*. Rifamycin binds and inhibits the essential β-subunit of RNA polymerase (RNAP). With regard to side effects, rifampicin (RIF) causes a red-orange staining of all body fluids, nausea, vomiting, diarrhea, and more infrequently, hepatitis and hypersensitivity reactions such as thrombocytopaenia, haemolytic anaemia and interstitial nephritis. Rare side effects include shock and hypotension, shortness of breath, organic brain syndrome and peripheral neurophathy [14].

Corticosteroid treatments are effective against T1R, however, neurological impairment persists in about 30-50% of cases [15]. Corticosteroids that bind the glucocorticoid receptor have been shown to suppress the expression of proinflammatory cytokines through NF-κB. [16-18].

Toll-like receptor 2 that recognizes diacylated lipopeptides (TLR2::TLR6) and triacylated lipopeptides (TLR1::TLR2), both common in mycobacteria, signals through MyD88 and IRAK, subsequently leading to NF-κB activation and production of hBDs [2] and LL-37 [19].

Thalidomide (N-a-phthalimidoglutarimide) inhibits NF-κB activation and inflammation [20]. However, thalidomide is a drug with well-known teratogenic effects [21]. Thalidomide was first applied as a sedative in the late 1950s, but the birth of more than ten thousand children with birth defects resulted in the withdrawal of it from the market in 1962. Thalidomide affects almost all organs of the fetus but the main defects are concentrated in ears, eyes, limbs and heart [22].

The fluoroquinolones (FQs) are important agents for the treatment of urinary tract infections, tuberculosis and leprosy. FQs comprise of ciprofloxacin, gemifloxacin, levofloxacin, moxifloxacin, norfloxacin and ofloxacin. FQs are believed to act by inhibiting type II DNA topoisomerases (gyrases) that are required for transcription of bacterial mRNA and DNA replication. In the latter, the use of FQs has enabled a dramatic shortening of formerly long and complicated therapy [23]. However, the common side effects of FQs are headaches, gastrointestinal disturbances, skin rashes and allergic reactions. Less common but more severe side effects include idiosyncratic liver injury (in a rate of 1:100,000 persons-exposed within 1-4 weeks of starting therapy), seizures, QT prolongation, hallucinations, tendon rupture, angioedema and photosensitivity (www.livertox.nlm.nih.gov).

The Role of Antimicrobial Peptides in Leprosy

Role of Defensins

There is increasing evidence that APs play an important role in leprosy. During T1Rs, hBD3 is significantly upregulated in the skin. Surprisingly, even though macrophages play a major role in leprosy pathogenesis, HaCaT keratinocytes but not macrophages upregulate hBD2 and hBD3 in response to nonviable sonicated *M. leprae in vitro* [2].

Also, the variation in defensin genes seems to be relevant in the severity instead of the susceptibility to disease. In a Mexican sample population the SNP rs1800972 (also called 668 or -44 C/G) in human β-defensin 1 (*DEFB1*) was associated with lepromatous leprosy. This SNP alters one out of five putative binding sites for NF-κB1 (p50/p105) in a small region of 0.5 kB of

5´UTR in *DEFB1*. We suggested that C allele in this locus render diminished constitutive expression and thus confer more permissiveness to *M. leprae* dissemination in patients already infected [24].

Role of Hepcidin

The *HAMP* gene encodes a propeptide of 84 amino acids that undergo enzymatic cleavage into mature peptides of 20, 22 and 25 amino acids [3], eight of them are cysteines that form 4 disulfide bridges [25]. Hepcidin is both a hormone and antimicrobial peptide that acts as a key regulator of iron absorption in mammals and it is considered an acute phase protein. In mice and cultured hepatocytes, IL-6 is the main mediator of iron-dependent hepcidin increment and this is the suggested cause of the hypoferremia in inflammation [26]. The hypoferremia is thought to increase host resistance to microbial infection but also leads to the anemia of inflammation (often referred to as the anemia of chronic disease) [27]. Upon activation of sensor Pattern Recognition Receptors (PPRs), secreted IL-6 induces hepcidin expression and release from the liver. In human monocytes (THP-1) LPS-induced hepcidin results bind directly to ferroportin [28] and induces its degradation [29]. Ferroportin is an iron exporter efflux protein on the surface of absortive intestinal enterocytes, macrophages, hepatocytes and placental cells, all of which release iron into plasma [27]. After ferroportin is degraded, firstly iron egresses from duodenal enterocytes and macrophages are diminished, resulting in hypoferremia as a host response to limit circulating iron availability to extracellular pathogens. Secondly, the protein kinase Jak2 becomes activated resulting in phosphorylation of not only ferroportin, but also the transcription factor Stat3 that induces transcriptional changes to modulate downstream acute cytokine-induced inflammatory responses [29]. Based on a mice model, the regulatory variation in hepcidin expression has been suggested as a heritable quantitative trait with the limitation that humans only have one hepcidin gene instead of two [30]. Another study in mice suggests that hepcidin upregulation is not necessary to induce anaemia by *M. avium* [31]. Although hepatocytes are the main source of hepcidin, in mice also is expressed in leukocytes mainly neutrophils and macrophages in response to Gram-positive (group A Streptococcus strain 5448) and Gram-negative bacteria (*Pseudomonas aeruginosa* ATCC 27853 and *Salmonella typhimurium* ATCC 13311) in a TLR4-dependent manner [32]. There is less information in humans, however, *M. tuberculosis* components as mannose-capped lipoarabinomannan and phosphatidyl-myo-inositol mannosides indeed upregulate hepcidin transcription in alveolar A549 epithelial cells [33].

Furthermore, in iron-depleted monocyte-derived macrophages (MDM´s) isolated from patients with mutations in hemochromatosis gene (*HFE*), *M. tuberculosis* growth was 50% less when compared with MDM controls [34].

Particularly in leprosy, hepcidin is present primarily in multibacillary (MB) lesions. In these patients decreases in total iron binding capacity and haematological parameters as haemoglobin, haematocrit, red blood cells count were observed [35].

Role of Cathelicidin LL-37

In *M. tuberculosis* infection, type I IFNs inhibit IL-1, a cytokine also required for the induction of vitamin D antimicrobial pathway [36] and the subsequent induction of cathelicidin LL-37 [19].

In this pathway, promoted by IL-15 the macrophages become less phagocytic [37]. In leprosy, type I IFN program is markedly upregulated in L-lep lesions and inhibits the IFN-γ-induced antimicrobial response against *M. leprae* in a IL-10-dependent fashion. In addition, type I IFNs block the ability of inflammasome activators. Serum levels of LL-37 are diminished in leprosy patients and the reduction is more marked in non-treated patients (untreated median=48 ng/mL *vs* treated median= 98 ng/mL). Furthermore, untreated patients were found to have an inverse correlation between serum vitamin D and LL-37 [38]. One possible explanation is the hypoxia-dependent cathelicidin upregulation in keratinocyte defense demonstrated in mice [39].

In *CAMP*, the human gene that codes for LL-37, we found several sites for hypoxia-inducible factor 1α (HIF-1α) and common SNPs (>1% in the population) alters them with potential impact in mycobacterial diseases [40, 41]. In leprosy, the diminished levels of LL-37 is probably mediated by micro RNA hsa-mir-21 that is upregulated in *M. leprae*-infected monocytes and causes inhibition of *CAMP* and *DEFB4* genes [42]. Notably, we recently found that cathelicidin gene is expressed constitutively in human normal keratinocytes (Flores Miramontes et al., submitted) reinforcing the concept that the keratinocyte is fundamental not only as mechanical barrier but as an innate immunity active site [43].

Antimicrobial Peptide Inhibitors As Potential Treatment of Leprosy

T1R often occurs after starting multidrug therapy (MDT) or during the puerperium [44]. During T1Rs, hBD3 is significantly up-regulated in the skin.

Also, keratinocytes but not macrophages up-regulate hBD2 and hBD3 in response to *M. leprae in vitro* [2]. There are at least 12 proinflammatory regulators of innate immunity that are up/downregulated in T1R [15]. The measure of these markers (Table 1) could help in analyze the effectivity of APIs and antimicrobial peptide elicitors (APEs) in leprosy. Antimicrobial peptide inhibitors (APIs) are agents that downregulate APs transcription [19, 45], Classification and effects of APIs are explained in table 2.

It has been suggested that hepcidin-mediated iron sequestration could promote *M. leprae* growth. In mice livers, hepcidin-suppressing molecules produced by Kupffer cells control body iron homeostasis independent of the iron-sensing molecule hemojuvelin [46]. Furthermore, in a rat model, small molecule dorsomorphin derivative LDN-193189 and protein soluble hemojuvelin-Fc (HJV.Fc) that inhibits hepcidin transcription are suggested as potential drugs to reverse anemia of chronic inflammation can also be useful to treat leprosy [47, 48]. Also, rationally designed minihepcidins with improved oral bioavailability and resistance to proteolysis diminish liver iron in mice [49]. Infectious microorganisms as *M. leprae* may acquire the ability to both evade immune surveillance and resist antibiotics, but it is less probable that they can escape their basic iron requirement for growth [25].

Iron supplementation may be futile (or even detrimental) in individuals with increased hepcidin, as the blockade of ferroportin likely prevents iron absortion and transport to bone marrow. Thus, to measure hepcidin could have prognostic value in leprosy [25]. For these reasons APIs of hepcidin could became the first drugs in regulating the iron metabolism pathway in leprosy.

Antimicrobial Peptide Elicitors As Potential Treatment of Leprosy

Even when LL-37 has been suggested as having potential in developing an antimycobacterial drug [47, 50] it is still expensive to produce peptides compared to the cost of conventional antibiotics [19, 49]. Furthermore, the *in vitro* resistance [51] and AP-induced pathogenicity by a PhoP-PhoQ-mediated system are additional drawbacks to use APs directly [52]. So there is a need for antimicrobial peptide elicitors (APE), which are defined as physical, chemical or biological agents that promote the upregulation of specific endogenous APs. [19].

Known signaling pathways of APEs are depicted in Figure 1.

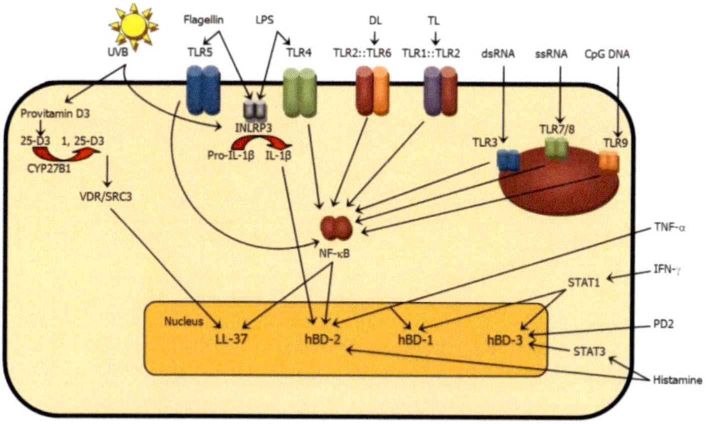

Taken from Prado Montes de Oca [19], ©Ernesto Prado Montes de Oca.

Figure 1. Pathways of APEs in human keratinocytes. From provitamin D3 (7-dehydrocholesterol), ultraviolet light B (UVB) produces the synthesis of calcidiol (25-hydroxy vitamin D3, 25,D3) and then by 25-hydroxyvitamin D3 1-α-hydroxylase 1 (CYP27B1) action, produces 1, 25-dyhydroxy vitamin D3 (1,25 D3), the active form of vitamin D. 1, 25 D3 binds and activates the vitamin D receptor (VDR) which recruits coactivator proteins. Activated VDR forms a complex with steroid receptor coactivator 3 (SRC3) leading to recruitment of histone acetyltransferases. Histone acetylation activates chromatin, presumably facilitating access to transcription machinery in *CAMP* gene producing LL-37 peptide, however, histone acetylation in *CAMP* promoter is still controversial, and an indirect activation through upregulation of transcription factors that bind *CAMP* promoter has been suggested. A second UVB-mediated APs expression pathway is through Inflammasome Nucleotide Oligomerization Domain-Like family, Pyrin domain-containing 3 (INLRP3). The activated caspase 1 of INLRP3 processes prointerleukin-1β (pro-IL-1 β) into biologically active IL-1β which is an elicitor of hBD-2. Psoriasin, hBD-1, hBD-2 and hBD-3 are also upregulated by UVB but whether this expression is VDR-dependent is unknown. Flagellin through Toll-like receptor 5 (TLR5), lipopolysaccharide (LPS) through TLR4, diacyllipopeptide (DL) through heterodimers composed of TLR2 and TLR6, triacyllipopeptide (TL) through heterodimers composed of TLR1 and TLR2 activates nuclear factor kappa B (NF-κB). In endosomes, dsRNA through TLR3, ssRNA through TLR7/8 and unmethylated CpG DNA through TLR9 also activates nuclear factor kappa B (NF-κB). NF-κB activation leads to LL-37 and hBD-2 expression. Psoriasin is upregulated through TLR5 probably by NF-κB pathway (not shown). LPS induces hBD-1 by an unknown pathway and hBD-2 through NF-κB.

In endosomes, TLR3, TLR7/8 and TLR9 also activate NF-κB. TNF-α induces upregulation of hBD-1 and hBD-2. IFN-γ through JAK-Signal Transducer and Activator of Transcription (STAT1) induces hBD-1, hBD-3. Prostaglandin D2 (PD2) upregulates hBD-3. Histamine induces hBD-2 and hBD-3, the latter through STAT3 (not shown). Detailed expression pathways for most APEs are unknown.

Classification, tissue-and gene-specificity of APEs are explained in table 2.

Elicitors of defensins. IL-10 is expressed in lepromatous leprosy (L-lep) lesions. This cytokine is an API of hBD-2, LL-37 [53] and probably of hBD-4 [54]. Conveniently, IL-10 is also an APE of hepcidin [55]. Theoretically a molecule that blocks the IL-10 could serve as useful APE in leprosy. As examples, IL-37 inhibits IL-10 in a HaCaT model of psoriasis [56] and the cytokine-suppresive anti-inflammatory drug (CSAID) N-acetyl cysteine (NAC) inhibits IL-10 in placental membrane [57]. However, caution must be sought because the predicted risks of excesive IL-10 inhibition is an increase in susceptibility to allergic rhinitis [58] and acute pyelonephritis [59] as well as probably other allergic disease and opportunistic infections.

Elicitors of LL-37. 1,25, dihidroxy-vitamin D3 (1,25-D3), the active form of vitamin D is a class II-A APE for the antimycobacterial genes *CAMP* (in macrophages and keratinocytes) and *DEFB4* (in macrophages) [19]. In leprosy, 1,25-D3 was successfully applied as therapeutic adjuvant [60]. 1,25-D3 enhances macrophage phagocytosis of *M. tuberculosis* inducing a LL-37-dependent autophagy and expression of beclin-1 and Atg5 [61]. Thus LL-37 has two different antimycobacterial functions: directly killing of mycobacteria and indirectly inducing autophagy [62]. Vitamin D also exerts is effects on several immune cell types, including dendritic cells (DCs), B and T cells. Vitamin D decreases the maturation of DCs and their production of pro-inflammatory cytokines and both directly and indirectly influences T_H cell differentiation. Also, vitamin D inhibits proliferation of B cells and antibody-secreting cells, and also inhibits both plasma cell differentiation and immunoglobulin production [63].

Noteworthy, polymorphisms in vitamin D receptor (VDR) have been associated with leprosy susceptibility, probably affecting the maturation of DCs and/or proliferation of B cells in these patients [64-68].

Table 1. Genes up/downregulated in type 1 reactions (T1Rs) of leprosy according to Orlova et al., [15] and their known function

Gene	Name	Fold Change	Function
ADA	Adenosine deaminase	1.39	Catalyzes the irreversible deamination of adenosine and deoxyadenosine in the purine catabolic pathway
CCL2	chemokine, CC motif, ligand 2	1.8	Previously called monocyte chemotactic protein-1 (MCP-1). Recruits monocytes to sites of injury and infection
CCL3	chemokine, CC motif, ligand 3 (macrophage inflammatory protein-1a)	1.36	Involved in the acute inflammatory state in the recruitment and activation of polymorphonuclear leukocytes
CCL3L1	chemokine, CC motif, ligand 3-like 1 (macrophage inflammatory protein-1aP)	1.35	Potent ligand for CCR5, a major coreceptor for macrophage-tropic, also called R5-tropic strains of HIV-1
CCL3L3	chemokine, CC motif, ligand 3-like 3	1.52	Centromeric copy of the CCL3L1 gene
CCL4L1	chemokine, CC motif, ligand 4-like 1 (lymphocyte activation gene 1, LAG1)	1.66	Directs the migration of specific subsets of leukocytes
CCL20	chemokine, CC motif, ligand 20 (macrophage inflammatory protein 3-alpha, MIP3A)	1.32	Ligand of CCR6
IL1A	Interleukin 1-alpha	1.47	Released after cell injury. Involved in apoptosis and inflammation
IL1B	Interleukin 1-beta	1.54	Endogenous pyrogen that mediates the acute phase response
IL6	Interleukin 6	1.33	Activates a cell surface signaling assembly composed of IL-6, IL6RA and the shared receptor gp130
IL23A	Interleukin 23-alpha	1.35	Enhances the IL-2-dependent secretion of IFNG by memory (CD45RO) but not naive (CD45RA) T cells. Key in autoiimune disorders as psoriasis
TNFAIP2	tumor necrosis factor-alpha-induced protein 2	0.71	Induced by TNF, IL1B and LPS
TAGAP	T-cell activation GTPase-activating protein	0.72	Expression peaks 4-6 h after T-cell activation. Coregulates with IL-2
FCAR	receptor for Fc fragment of IgA	0.73	Mediates phagocytosis, Ab-dependent cell-mediated toxicity and stimulation of the release of inflammatory mediators

Table 2. Classification of antimicrobial peptide elicitors (APEs) and inhibitors (APIs) and their effects on selected human antimicrobial peptides in different tissues and cell lines

					G	E	N	E	
Class	Subclass	Elicitor							
			CAMP LL-37	*DEFB1* hBD-1	*DEFB4* hBD-2	*DEFB103* hBD-3	*DEFB104* hBD-4	*HAMP* Hepcidin	*S100A7* Psoriasin
I. Physical	A. Light	UVB	K	HaCaT	SK, HaCaT	SK			SK
		UVA1 320-400 nm		SLS skin		SLS skin			
		UVA1		SUS skin		SUS skin			
II. Chemical	A. Vitamins	Vitamin D3/analogs	Mϕ, PK		Mo; PK	PK			PK
	B. Nucleicacids	Oligonucleotides CpG/RNA	K		BL; CEC, K				
	C. AA/proteins	Amino acids		HCT-116					
		Interleukins IL-1 α	Caco-2, HCA-7		HDP, AGS, As, RTC, HT29, CaCo-2, K				
		IL-1 β		MKN7	CEC, AGS, MKN7, As, GK, AE				
		IL-17	PPS; Mo		AEC; ADK; Mo				
		IFN-γ	Caco-2, HCA-7; Mo	GK	Mo	GK, ECUC, AEC, HaCaT, LS174T	LS174T		MDA-MB-468
		TNF-α		HaCaT	HDP, CEC,GK, AEC, HaCaT	LS174T	LS174T		
		Transcription factors p53		IS				HC	

					G	E	N	E	
Class	Subclass	Elicitor							
			CAMP LL-37	*DEFB1* hBD-1	*DEFB4* hBD-2	*DEFB103* hBD-3	*DEFB104* hBD-4	*HAMP* Hepcidin	*S100A7* Psoriasin
II. Chemical		AP-1	IS	IS	PEC, OE21, K	IS / OE21, K			
		NF-κB	HeLa, HaCaT, PK / IS	IS	CaCo2, PEC, OE21, K	K			
		c-Myc		HCT-116, HEK-293					
		Hormones Leptin			EK			HuH7	
		Insulin		HEK-293, HCT-116					
		Progesterone/ 17-β estradiol		IS	VEC				
		BSA		HCT-116					
		Salivarygland 100-kDa protein							
		Histamine			EK	EK			
	D. Carbohydrates	Glucose		HEK-293, HCT-116					
	E.Fatty acids and prebiotics	Sodium butyrate	CaCo2, HCA-7, HT-29		GEC				
		4-phenyl butyrate		VA10 / U937					
		Lithocholicacid	HT-29						
		Lauric/oleic/ palmitic acids			Seb				
III. Biological	A.Bacterial	Bacterial lysates			NM				
		E. coli		EPM	RTC, CaCo-2				
		H. pylori			AGS, MKN7		GE		

Table 2. (Continued)

					G	E	N	E	
Class	Subclass	Elicitor							
			CAMP LL-37	*DEFB1* hBD-1	*DEFB4* hBD-2	*DEFB103* hBD-3	*DEFB104* hBD-4	*HAMP* Hepcidin	*S100A7* Psoriasin
III. Biological		Bacterial exotoxins		Plat; IEC					
		Bacterial lipoprotein			HEK293, A549				
		LPS	Caco-2, HCA-7	GE C(1690), HaCaT; GE (1435/9)	As, HeLa, PKE6/E7, IEC, RE, LC2/ad, UEC, seb, A549 through MM6, hTBE, GE (1690), AMϕ, GK, HaCaT; GE (1435/9)	RE, OSCC, GE (1690); GE (1435/9)			
		Flagellin	HCEC		HCEC, K, CaCo2				EVSM, EK
	B.Plant	Crude extract			A549; T24, 5637				
	C.Fungal	Allergen	NTE						
	D.Mycobacteria	*Mycobacterium bovis*-BCG		PEC	PEC			PBMC	
	E.Virus	HIV		AMϕ	OEC, MDOE	OEC			
		PR8, HSV-1, Sendai virus		pDC, Mo					

	Upregulation			In silico transcriptional impact		
	Downregulation			Unknown		No effect

Modified from Prado Montes de Oca [19], ©Ernesto Prado Montes de Oca.

AP genes (italics) codify for the following peptides: *CAMP*, LL-37; *DEFB1*, hBD-1; *DEFB4*, hBD-2; *DEFB103*, hBD-3; *DEFB104*, hBD-4; *HAMP*, hepcidin; *S100A7*, psoriasin. 5637, primary bladder grade II carcinoma from an adult male patient; A549, human lung transformed epithelial cell line; 5637, grade II primary bladder carcinoma; ADK, atopic dermatitis keratinocytes; AEC, airway epithelium cells; AGS, human gastric adenocarcinoma cell line ATCC CRL 1739; AMϕ, alveolar macrophages; AP-1, activator protein 1; As, astrocytes; BL, B lymphocytes; BSA, bovine serum albumin; CaCo-2, colon carcinoma cells; CEC, corneal epithelial cells; C-myc, cellular V-myc avian myelocytomatosis viral oncogene homolog; ECUC; epidermal cell of ulcerative colitis; EK, epithelial keratinocytes; EPM, extraplacental membranes; EVSM, extravascular smooth muscle cells; GEC, gastric epithelium cells; GK, gingival keratinocytes; GM-CSF, granulocyte/monocyte-colony stimulating factor; HaCaT, human adult low calcium high temperature keratinocyte cell line; HC, hepatoma cells; HCA7, colon carcinoma cell line; HCEC, human corneal epithelial cells; HCT-116, human colon cells; HDP, human dental pulp; HEK-293; human epithelial kidney cells; HeLa, cervical uterine cancer cell line; HSG, human salivary gland; HSV-1, herpes simplex virus-1; HT29, human colon grade II adenocarcinoma; HTBE, human tracheobronchial epithelial cell; HuH7, hepatocellular carcinoma; IEC, human endothelial cells; IS, *in silico* approach; K, keratinocyte; LC2/ad, pulmonary adenocarcinoma; LS174T, human Caucasian colon adenocarcinoma; MDA-MB-468, breast cancer cell line; MDOE, multilayered differentiated oral epithelia; Mϕ, macrophage; MKN-7, human gastric carcinoma; Mo, monocytes; MM6, mono mac 6, human monocytic cell line from acute leukemia; NM, nasal mucosa; NTE, nasal tissue explants; OEC, oral epithelia cells; OE21, caucasic oesophageal squamous cell carcinoma; OSCC, oral squamous cell carcinoma; PBMC, peripheral blood mononuclear cells; Plat, platelets; pDC, plasmacitoid dendritic cells; PEC, pulmonary epithelial cells; PK, psoriatic keratinocyte; PKE6/E7, mutants derived from proximal kidney tubule cell line; PPS, psoriasis patient serum; PR8, influenza A virus, PR8 strain; RE, reticuloendothelial cells; RTC, renal epithelial tubular cells; Seb, sebocytes; SK, skin keratinocyte; SLS, sclerodermal lesional skin; SUS, sclerodermal unaffected skin, T24, grade III human urinary bladder carcinoma; U937, human leukemic monocyte lymphoma; UEC, uterine epithelial cells;VA10, bronquial epithelial cell line; VEC, vascular endothelial cells.

Conclusion

Antimicrobial peptide elicitors/inhibitors represent new molecules that can be useful in the treatment of leprosy specifically limiting *M. leprae* growth and prevent nerve damage in leprosy patients mainly due to the mediators present in T1R. Specifically, APIs that downregulate hepcidin could limit the iron availability of the pathogen and thus restrain *M. leprae* growth.

Additionally, APEs that upregulate the antimycobacterial LL-37 and hBDs could be beneficial to the treatment of leprosy and applied with theoretically lessened induction to side effects. However, the safety and efficacy issues *in vivo* of these new molecules in order to substitute or complement current therapies will be the next challenge to overcome.

Acknowledgments

Thanks to Tina Coop (Peace Corps) and Adolfo Flores (CIATEJ AC) for reviewing the manuscript. This work was supported by Fondos Mixtos del Gobierno del Estado de Aguascalientes-CONACYT (grant number AGS-2010-C02-143938). EPM receive a research stimulus from the Sistema Nacional de Investigadores (SNI 41290, CONACYT).

The sponsors had no involvement in the writing of the manuscript or in the decision to submit the manuscript for publication.

References

[1] Prado Montes de Oca, E., Human polymorphisms as clinical predictors in leprosy. *Journal of tropical medicine*, 2011. 2011: p. 923943.

[2] Cogen, A. L., et al., Human beta-defensin 3 is up-regulated in cutaneous leprosy type 1 reactions. *PLoS neglected tropical diseases*, 2012. 6: p. e1869.

[3] Park, C. H., et al., Hepcidin, a urinary antimicrobial peptide synthesized in the liver. *The Journal of biological chemistry*, 2001. 276: p. 7806-10.

[4] Li, W., et al., Real-time PCR and high-resolution melt analysis for rapid detection of Mycobacterium leprae drug resistance mutations and strain types. *Journal of clinical microbiology*, 2012. 50: p. 742-53.

[5] Singh, P., et al., Genome-wide re-sequencing of multidrug-resistant Mycobacterium leprae Airaku-3. *Clinical microbiology and infection: the official publication of the European Society of Clinical Microbiology and Infectious Diseases*, 2014. DOI 10.1111/1469-0691.12609

[6] Deps, P., et al., Hemolytic anemia in patients receiving daily dapsone for the treatment of leprosy. *Leprosy review*, 2012. 83: p. 305-7.

[7] Dupnik, K. M., et al., Intolerance to leprosy multi-drug therapy: more common in women? *Leprosy review*, 2013. 84: p. 209-18.

[8] Schalcher, T. R., et al., Clinical oxidative stress during leprosy multidrug therapy: impact of dapsone oxidation. *PLoS One*, 2014. 9: p. e85712.

[9] Grosset, J. H., T. G. Singer and W. R. Bishai, New drugs for the treatment of tuberculosis: hope and reality. *The international journal of tuberculosis and lung disease: the official journal of the International Union against Tuberculosis and Lung Disease,* 2012. 16: p. 1005-14.

[10] Maia, M. V., G. Cunha Mda and C. S. Cunha, Adverse effects of alternative therapy (minocycline, ofloxacin, and clofazimine) in multibacillary leprosy patients in a recognized health care unit in Manaus, Amazonas, Brazil. *Anais brasileiros de dermatologia*, 2013. 88: p. 205-10.

[11] Singh, H., K. Azad and K. Kaur, Clofazimine-induced enteropathy in a patient of leprosy. *Indian journal of pharmacology*, 2013. 45: p. 197-8.

[12] Lorenz, M., G. Wozel and J. Schmitt, Hypersensitivity reactions to dapsone: a systematic review. *Acta dermato-venereologica*, 2012. 92: p. 194-9.

[13] Zhang, F. R., et al., HLA-B*13:01 and the dapsone hypersensitivity syndrome. *The New England journal of medicine*, 2013. 369: p. 1620-8.

[14] Boeree, M. J., Rifamycins revisited, In: *Tuberculosis: laboratory diagnosis and treatment strategies 2013*, CAB International Croydon, UK.

[15] Orlova, M., et al., Gene set signature of reversal reaction type I in leprosy patients. *PLoS genetics*, 2013. 9: p. e1003624.

[16] Rao, N. A., et al., Coactivation of GR and NFKB alters the repertoire of their binding sites and target genes. *Genome research*, 2011. 21: p. 1404-16.

[17] Foteinou, P. T., et al., In silico simulation of corticosteroids effect on an NFkB- dependent physicochemical model of systemic inflammation. *PLoS One*, 2009. 4: p. e4706.

[18] Unlap, T. and R. S. Jope, Inhibition of NFkB DNA binding activity by glucocorticoids in rat brain. *Neuroscience letters*, 1995. 198: p. 41-4.

[19] Prado Montes de Oca, E., Antimicrobial Peptide Elicitors: new hope for the post-antibiotic era. *Innate Immun.*, 2013. 19: p. 227-41.

[20] Hernandez Mde, O., et al., Thalidomide modulates Mycobacterium leprae-induced NF-kappaB pathway and lower cytokine response. *European journal of pharmacology*, 2011. 670: p. 272-9.

[21] Ito, T., H. Ando and H. Handa, Teratogenic effects of thalidomide: molecular mechanisms. *Cellular and molecular life sciences: CMLS*, 2011. 68: p. 1569-79.

[22] Vianna, F. S., et al., Recognition of the phenotype of thalidomide embryopathy in countries endemic for leprosy: new cases and review of the main dysmorphological findings. *Clinical dysmorphology*, 2013. 22: p. 59-63.

[23] Rubinstein, E. and Y. Keynan, Quinolones for mycobacterial infections. *International journal of antimicrobial agents*, 2013. 42: p. 1-4.

[24] Prado-Montes de Oca, E., et al., SNP 668C (-44) alters a NF-kappaB1 putative binding site in non-coding strand of human beta-defensin 1 (DEFB1) and is associated with lepromatous leprosy. *Infection, genetics and evolution: journal of molecular epidemiology and evolutionary genetics in infectious diseases*, 2009. 9: p. 617-25.

[25] Drakesmith, H. and A. M. Prentice, Hepcidin and the iron-infection axis. *Science*, 2012. 338: p. 768-72.

[26] Nemeth, E., et al., IL-6 mediates hypoferremia of inflammation by inducing the synthesis of the iron regulatory hormone hepcidin. *The Journal of clinical investigation,* 2004. 113: p. 1271-6.

[27] Nemeth, E., et al., Hepcidin regulates cellular iron efflux by binding to ferroportin and inducing its internalization. *Science*, 2004. 306: p. 2090-3.

[28] Theurl, I., et al., Autocrine formation of hepcidin induces iron retention in human monocytes. *Blood*, 2008. 111: p. 2392-9.

[29] Johnson, E. E. and M. Wessling-Resnick, Iron metabolism and the innate immune response to infection. *Microbes and infection / Institut Pasteur,* 2012. 14: p. 207-16.

[30] Bayele, H. K. and S. K. Srai, Regulatory variation in hepcidin expression as a heritable quantitative trait. *Biochemical and biophysical research communications,* 2009. 384: p. 22-7.

[31] Rodrigues, P. N., et al., Mycobacteria-induced anaemia revisited: a molecular approach reveals the involvement of NRAMP1 and lipocalin-2, but not of hepcidin. *Immunobiology*, 2011. 216: p. 1127-34.

[32] Peyssonnaux, C., et al., TLR4-dependent hepcidin expression by myeloid cells in response to bacterial pathogens. *Blood*, 2006. 107: p. 3727-32.

[33] Sow, F. B., et al., Mycobacterium tuberculosis components stimulate production of the antimicrobial peptide hepcidin. *Tuberculosis*, 2011. 91: p. 314-21.

[34] Olakanmi, O., L. S. Schlesinger and B. E. Britigan, Hereditary hemochromatosis results in decreased iron acquisition and growth by Mycobacterium tuberculosis within human macrophages. *Journal of leukocyte biology*, 2007. 81: p. 195-204.

[35] Souza, V. N., et al., Increased hepcidin expression in multibacillary leprosy. *Memorias do Instituto Oswaldo Cruz, 2012*. 107 Suppl. 1: p. 183-9.

[36] Teles, R. M., et al., Type I interferon suppresses type II interferon-triggered human anti-mycobacterial responses. *Science*, 2013. 339: p. 1448-53.

[37] Montoya, D. and R. L. Modlin, Learning from leprosy: insight into the human innate immune response. *Advances in immunology*, 2010. 105: p. 1-24.

[38] Matzner, M., et al., Low serum levels of cathelicidin LL-37 in leprosy. *Acta tropica*, 2011. 117: p. 56-9.

[39] Peyssonnaux, C., et al., Critical role of HIF-1alpha in keratinocyte defense against bacterial infection. *The Journal of investigative dermatology,* 2008. 128: p. 1964-8.

[40] Lopez Campos, G. N., et al., Polymorphism in cathelicidin gene (CAMP) that alters Hypoxia-inducible factor (HIF-1alpha::ARNT) binding is not associated with tuberculosis. *International journal of immunogenetics,* 2014. 41: p. 54-62.

[41] Flores-Saiffe Farías, A., et al., Novel method to predict functional regulatory SNPs in human genes with an application on antimicrobial peptides in tuberculosis and HIV/AIDS (submitted).

[42] Liu, P. T., et al., MicroRNA-21 targets the vitamin D-dependent antimicrobial pathway in leprosy. *Nature medicine*, 2012. 18: p. 267-73.

[43] Schroder, J. M., The role of keratinocytes in defense against infection. *Current opinion in infectious diseases*, 2010. 23: p. 106-10.

[44] Prado Montes de Oca, E., Human beta defensin 1 (DEFB1) polymorphisms in leprosy susceptibility, PhD thesis*Human Genetics Department 2007,* Guadalajara University,. p. 75.

[45] Prado-Montes de Oca, E., Human beta-defensin 1: a restless warrior against allergies, infections and cancer. *Int. J. Biochem. Cell. Biol.*, 2010. 42: p. 800-4.

[46] Theurl, M., et al., Kupffer cells modulate iron homeostasis in mice via regulation of hepcidin expression. *Journal of molecular medicine*, 2008. 86: p. 825-35.

[47] Padhi, A., et al., Antimicrobial peptides and proteins in mycobacterial therapy: Current status and future prospects. *Tuberculosis*, 2014.

[48] Theurl, I., et al., Pharmacologic inhibition of hepcidin expression reverses anemia of chronic inflammation in rats. *Blood*, 2011. 118: p. 4977-84.

[49] Preza, G. C., et al., Minihepcidins are rationally designed small peptides that mimic hepcidin activity in mice and may be useful for the treatment of iron overload. *The Journal of clinical investigation*, 2011. 121: p. 4880-8.

[50] Mendez-Samperio, P., The human cathelicidin hCAP18/LL-37: a multifunctional peptide involved in mycobacterial infections. *Peptides*, 2010. 31(9): p. 1791-8.

[51] Perron, G. G., M. Zasloff and G. Bell, Experimental evolution of resistance to an antimicrobial peptide. Proceedings. *Biological sciences / The Royal Society,* 2006. 273: p. 251-6.

[52] Prost, L. R., et al., The PhoQ histidine kinases of Salmonella and Pseudomonas spp. are structurally and functionally different: evidence that pH and antimicrobial peptide sensing contribute to mammalian pathogenesis. *Molecular microbiology*, 2008. 69: p. 503-19.

[53] Howell, M. D., et al., Interleukin-10 downregulates anti-microbial peptide expression in atopic dermatitis. *The Journal of investigative dermatology,* 2005. 125: p. 738-45.

[54] Dreno, B., et al., Hidradenitis suppurativa: the role of deficient cutaneous innate immunity. *Archives of dermatology*, 2012. 148: p. 182-6.

[55] Huang, H., et al., Interleukin-10 regulates hepcidin in Plasmodium falciparum malaria. *PLoS One*, 2014. 9: p. e88408.

[56] Teng, X., et al., IL-37 ameliorates the inflammatory process in psoriasis by suppressing proinflammatory cytokine production. *Journal of immunology,* 2014. 192: p. 1815-23.

[57] Stinson, L. F., et al., Effects of cytokine-suppressive anti-inflammatory drugs on inflammatory activation in ex vivo human and ovine fetal membranes. *Reproduction*, 2014. 147: p. 313-20.

[58] Wang, S. B., et al., Exogenous interleukin-10 alleviates allergic inflammation but inhibits local interleukin-10 expression in a mouse allergic rhinitis model. *BMC immunology*, 2014. 15: p. 9.
[59] Javor, J., et al., Association of interleukin-10 gene promoter polymorphisms with susceptibility to acute pyelonephritis in children. *Folia microbiologica*, 2014.
[60] Herrera, G., Vitamin D in massive doses as an adjuvant to the sulfones in the treatment of tuberculoid leprosy. *International journal of Leprosy*, 1949. 17: p. 35-42.
[61] Selvaraj, P., Vitamin D, vitamin D receptor, and cathelicidin in the treatment of tuberculosis. *Vitamins and hormones*, 2011. 86: p. 307-25.
[62] Yuk, J. M., et al., Vitamin D3 induces autophagy in human monocytes/macrophages via cathelicidin. *Cell host and microbe*, 2009. 6: p. 231-43.
[63] Veldhoen, M. and V. Brucklacher-Waldert, Dietary influences on intestinal immunity. Nature reviews. *Immunology*, 2012. 12: p. 696-708.
[64] Sapkota, B. R., et al., Association of TNF, MBL, and VDR polymorphisms with leprosy phenotypes. *Human immunology*, 2010. 71: p. 992-8.
[65] Goulart, L. R., F. R. Ferreira and I. M. Goulart, Interaction of TaqI polymorphism at exon 9 of the vitamin D receptor gene with the negative lepromin response may favor the occurrence of leprosy. *FEMS immunology and medical microbiology,* 2006. 48: p. 91-8.
[66] Roy, S., et al., Association of vitamin D receptor genotype with leprosy type. *The Journal of infectious diseases*, 1999. 179: p. 187-91.
[67] Velarde Felix, J. S., et al., Association between the TaqI polymorphism of the vitamin D receptor gene and lepromatous leprosy in a Mexican population sample. *Salud Publica de Mexico*, 2009. 51: p. 59-61.
[68] Fitness, J., et al., Large-scale candidate gene study of leprosy susceptibility in the Karonga district of northern Malawi. *The American journal of tropical medicine and hygiene,* 2004. 71: p. 330-40.

Index

#

A

D

E

F

G

H

I

K

L

M

N

O

R

S

T

U

V

W

Y